PRACTICAL LECTURES IN PSYCHIATRY FOR THE MEDICAL PRACTITIONER

PRACTICAL LECTURES IN PSYCHIATRY FOR THE MEDICAL PRACTITIONER

Edited by

GENE L. USDIN, M.D.

Chief, Division of Neurology and Psychiatry
Touro Infirmary
New Orleans, Louisiana

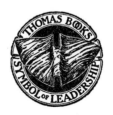

CHARLES C THOMAS • PUBLISHER
Springfield • Illinois • U.S.A.

Published and Distributed Throughout the World by

CHARLES C THOMAS • PUBLISHER

BANNERSTONE HOUSE

301-327 East Lawrence Avenue, Springfield, Illinois, U.S.A.

NATCHEZ PLANTATION HOUSE

735 North Atlantic Boulevard, Fort Lauderdale, Florida, U.S.A.

© *1966, by* CHARLES C THOMAS • PUBLISHER

Library of Congress Catalog Card Number: 66-12452

*With THOMAS BOOKS careful attention is given to all details of
manufacturing and design. It is the Publisher's desire to present books
that are satisfactory as to their physical qualities and artistic possibilities
and appropriate for their particular use. THOMAS BOOKS will be true
to those laws of quality that assure a good name and good will.*

Printed in the United States of America

W-2

LIST OF CONTRIBUTORS

ARTHUR P. BURDON, M.D.

Junior Associate, Division of Neurology and Psychiatry
Touro Infirmary
Associate Professor of Clinical Psychiatry
Louisiana State University School of Medicine
New Orleans, Louisiana

ALVIN COHEN, M.D.

Senior, Division of Neurology and Psychiatry
Touro Infirmary
Associate Professor of Clinical Psychiatry
Louisiana State University School of Medicine
New Orleans, Louisiana

MAYO EMORY, M.D.

Senior, Department of Internal Medicine
Touro Infirmary
New Orleans, Louisiana

JACK EWALT, M.D.

Professor of Psychiatry, Harvard Medical School
Past President, American Psychiatric Association
Boston, Massachusetts

DONALD GALLANT, M.D.

Associate Professor of Psychiatry
Tulane Medical School
New Orleans, Louisiana

EDWARD H. KNIGHT, M.D.

Senior, Division of Neurology and Psychiatry
Touro Infirmary
Associate Professor of Clinical Psychiatry
Louisiana State University School of Medicine
New Orleans, Louisiana

JAMES A. KNIGHT, M.D.

Assistant Dean, Tulane School of Medicine
Consultant, Division of Neurology and Psychiatry
Touro Infirmary
New Orleans, Louisiana

JOHN LAMBERT, M.D.

Medical Director, Four Winds Hospital, Katonah, New York
Chairman, Committee on Private Practice and Psychiatry
American Psychiatric Association

ZIGMOND LEBENSOHN, M.D.

Chief, Department of Psychiatry
Sibley Memorial Hospital, Washington, D. C.
Clinical Professor of Psychiatry
Georgetown University School of Medicine
Washington, D. C.

IRWIN M. MARCUS, M.D.

Senior Associate, Division of Neurology and Psychiatry
Touro Infirmary
Professor of Clinical Psychiatry
Louisiana State University School of Medicine
New Orleans, Louisiana

MARSHALL L. MICHEL, M.D.

Chief, Division of Surgery
Touro Infirmary
Associate Professor of Clinical Psychiatry
Tulane Medical School
New Orleans, Louisiana

PHILIP SOLOMON, M.D.

Chairman, Committee on Medical Practice
American Psychiatric Association
Associate Professor of Clinical Psychiatry
Harvard Medical School
Physician-in-Chief for Psychiatry
Boston City Hospital
Boston, Massachusetts

WILLIAM R. SORUM, M.D.

Senior Associate, Division of Neurology and Psychiatry
Touro Infirmary
Assistant Professor of Clinical Psychiatry
Tulane Medical School
New Orleans, Louisiana

ERNEST O. SVENSON, M.D.

Junior Associate, Division of Neurology and Psychiatry
Touro Infirmary
Assistant Professor of Clinical Psychiatry
Louisiana State University School of Medicine
New Orleans, Louisiana

MOTTRAM TORRE, M.D.

Clinical Assistant, Division of Neurology and Psychiatry
Touro Infirmary
Lecturer, Department of Psychiatry and Neurology
and
Lecturer, Department of Public Health and Tropical Medicine
Tulane Medical School
New Orleans, Louisiana

TED A. WATTERS, M.D.

Professor of Clinical Psychiatry
Louisiana State University School of Medicine
New Orleans, Louisiana

THOMAS G. WEBSTER, M.D.

Training Specialist in Psychiatry
National Institute of Mental Health
Bethesda, Maryland

WILLIAM S. WIEDORN, M.D.

Senior Associate, Division of Neurology and Psychiatry
Touro Infirmary
Assistant Professor of Clinical Psychiatry
Louisiana State University School of Medicine
New Orleans, Louisiana

This volume is dedicated to Touro Infirmary which even before the Civil War served "both white and slave" and which today continues to maintain leadership in research, medical education and service to the entire community.

G. L. U.

PREFACE

THE COMPLEXITY OF medical practice continues to increase for busy practitioners, and the increase goes by an exponential rate. The range and abundance of new knowledge in medicine all but overwhelm the individual intelligence. The impact of population growth, the lowered mortality rate, the increasing life span, and the intellectual and economic upgrading of an entire population have brought patients and patient needs in vastly increasing numbers to the offices, clinics, and hospitals of a physician population which is increasing nowhere proportionately as fast. The inevitable result in many cases is continuously rising graphs for average patient loads, hours of practice, and types of cases seen. The physician often experiences a feeling of futility in trying to keep abreast.

Often, as a consequence, he wants to restrict himself to a specialty or to circumscribe his practice in some manner. He is likely to find himself yearning for a time when he was not overwhelmed by the rapid introduction of new drugs and techniques and when periodicals and books were not so inundating, so enriched, and so formidably competent. He may recognize the necessity of attending courses, lectures, and symposia, some of which may be a considerable distance from where he lives, all the while realizing that he cannot spare the time away from his practice. Because he deals primarily with treating people, he is more acutely involved with the dilemma of our times—maintaining his maximum potential in actual practice in the face of an unavoidable obligation to read, attend, study, and reflect on the torrential flow of professional, factual knowledge.

Probably no field of medicine has undergone such tremendous growth as psychiatry. The practice of psychiatry bears little resemblance to what it was before the second World War. Factual information has increased enormously, and techniques have changed dramatically. Dynamic concepts of the conscious and unconscious have become an integral part of the modern medical outlook. The necessity for an eclectic approach has become more evident, and fortunately there has been less conflict between proponents of physical techniques (drugs, electric treatments, etc.) and proponents of psychological techniques (psychotherapy) and vice versa. There is emerging a more consistent framework for medical practitioners to utilize. It is an interesting commentary that psychiatry now is outranked only by internal medicine and surgery in the number of residents taking training.

Mental health is being recognized as a national resource, and nonpsychiatric physicians have increasingly assumed a role in helping to educate the general public regarding mental health and illness. Medical practitioners, whether they be dermatologists, internists, pediatricians, general practitioners or in any other field of medicine, have become increasingly aware of the influence of the emotions on their patients.

The advent of the newer psychopharmacologic drugs has provided a forum where psychiatrists and nonpsychiatrists can have a common meeting ground. Each can learn from the other regarding the effects of drugs and especially how these drugs can be utilized in their practices. With the increased number of psychiatrists, more psychiatrists are around hospital corridors and nonpsychiatrists develop personal contacts whereby they can better understand the problems of psychiatry and also realize that the psychiatrist is not the eccentric, unreal person which society has painted him in the past.

One of the most dramatic developments has been the attempt by medical practitioners to learn more about psychiatry and its techniques not only to better understand and help their patients but also to assist patients in getting specialized help when indicated. The number of symposia, institutes, and courses in the past ten years has multiplied together with increased attendance and interest. The American Medical Association and the American Psychiatric Association have taken cognizance of this need for post-graduate education in psychiatry for non-psychiatric physicians. The National Institute of Mental Health has been particularly active in this area.

The Division of Neurology and Psychiatry of Touro Infirmary, in an effort to respond to this growing need of the medical practitioner for post-graduate education in psychiatry, sponsored a symposium March 4, 5, 6, 1965, in New Orleans. This symposium was supported by Public Health Service Training Grant No. T1-MH 8593-01, from the Training and Manpower Resources Branch, National Institute of Mental Health. Emphasis was not on esoteric theoretical concepts but rather on knowledge and practical techniques that would be suitable for the nonpsychiatrist. Speakers attempted to be as clinically oriented and practical as possible. Four panels followed by audience participation were held during the symposium and audience participation proved to be active and provocative. This volume is the content of the proceedings of the two-and-a-half-day symposium.

GENE L. USDIN, M.D.

CONTENTS

PRACTICAL LECTURES IN PSYCHIATRY FOR THE MEDICAL PRACTITIONER

TREATMENT OF EMOTIONAL STATES BY THE MEDICAL PRACTITIONER

MAYO L. EMORY, M.D.

EUCRASIA:* OR THE WELL-TEMPERED HUMAN

To a healthy man everything seems healthy.
RUSSIAN PROVERB

EUCRASIA MEANS THE "normal state of health," or "physical well-being." It comes from the Greek term meaning well-tempered, and this raises an interesting question: What factors lead to eucrasia—absence of disease alone or the frame of mind?

In a brief report, Asher (1) describes a ninety-year-old woman who has been busy at work for seventy-six consecutive years. With only ten days' illness in 1932, she has been both cook and housekeeper for a girls' day school for forty-two years. Her work is strenuous and responsible and includes cooking for ninety people, shopping, cleaning, polishing, washing, and also walking her dog at 6:30 a.m. and 1 p.m.

This alert, spry little woman enjoys her work. (She also "never consults doctors.") Now, although her good fortune is probably a hereditary gift (her mother lived to be 100, and three siblings are over age eighty-six), one wonders how much significance lies in this brief phrase, "she enjoys her work." The experience of most of us would lead us to believe that "physical well-being" is more positive than (the negative) "absence of illness." Certainly, we have felt buoyant and exhilarated, but we have also felt merely "O.K." at times when we have had no

---

* *Physicians Bulletin,* Vol. XXII, No. 6, p. 71-72, Aug. 15, 1958. By permission Eli Lilly Co.

3

detectable illness. Perhaps these variations in eucrasia are due to sunspots, to barometric pressure, or to more personal matters. The fundamental question seems to be: Do you feel happy, optimistic, alert, and vigorous because your organic health is good, or is your physical state "good" because you enjoy your work and your life?

Is this the paradox of the chicken and the egg? Perhaps the truth, as far as man can know it, lies in the Greek origin of eucrasia, the well-tempered.

> The sound body is the product of the
> sound mind.   G. B. SHAW

I shall not presume to tell you how you should treat or handle patients with emotional states or illness. However, I will tell you how I meet these problems, why I choose to tackle them, and how I select the patients I shall treat, refer, or reject. Maybe this will be helpful to you, maybe you will find attitudes you will wish to adopt, to reject, or to modify.

First, I assume that all patients and all persons have emotional problems. I presume that many people are perfectly capable of coping with their problems, that some people don't want me to monkey with their emotional processes, some people sincerely want advice, help, reassurance, or a chance to air their problems, and some are dying to tell me all about themselves. Second, I assume that I am a trained physician, that I am attentive, observant, and that I am capable of meeting personal problems, of advising, of referring, or of declining to undertake a case. Third, I respect my patient no matter how perverse, silly, aggravating, pleasant, beautiful, or wealthy. Fourth, I expect the patient to respect me and the people with whom I work. All of these transactions take place without any formal exchange but the point gets across by my attitude and the attitude of my office and hospital workers.

I further assume that I am honest and that I can speak forthrightly without offending the patient or harming myself. I also assume that the patient may not be honest with me, that he may try to manipulate me, use me, or bald-facedly lie to me. He may misinterpret purposefully or innocently. He may flatter me, love me, and try to demolish me. Therefore, I am wary, contemplative, and observant but not necessarily suspicious.

In short, I would like to say I am not afraid of patients. I am not afraid of harming them, using them, or failing them. I frankly like the practice of medicine, its challenges, its dangers, its subtleties and therein lies the joy of practice.

I believe the greatest diagnostic tool at my command is my ear. To listen attentively, to observe closely, and to prod appropriately requires my entire mind. I also believe that the ear is *your* greatest therapeutic tool—it is the gateway to understanding. Listening to the patient is only part of the process. I am a firm believer that a careful and detailed physical examination is an integral part of treatment. When you have carefully examined a patient and you can look him in the eye and tell him you do not find trouble or you do need more studies, he knows you are not talking through your hat. When you can examine a woman's breast or do a pelvic examination without embarrassment, you have conveyed a message. When you have proctoscoped a patient gently and thoroughly, the patient knows you have really looked inside. To have proctoscoped him otherwise has told him something in addition. To touch a patient is important; it conveys a message to me and my touch conveys a message to the patient. The touch of the healer has been recognized since time immemorial as the therapeutic ritual of all cultures.

By my actions I imply that I am responsible and will be responsible for the course of action we, the patient and I, are to undertake or to explore. I tell the patient that I understand and that I shall try to help, or that I do not understand, or that I am not competent to help him but that I will try to get him into the proper hands. I promise nothing except to work within the bounds of my competence and to seek help when and where I need it.

So much for my approach.

What about the patient? Well, I cannot accept the dichotomy of mind and body or of body and soul. To me a patient is a biological phenomenon with that most complex of biologic attributes, mind. That the brain is the organ of the mind and that the mind is all-important and pervades the entire organism is to me self-evident. That the brain can be disordered is to me not remarkable. That it is not more frequently disordered is to me always amazing. That disorder of the brain or the information that is fed to the brain and consequently the interaction of the brain with this information should be reflected in disorder of the mind or that the mind should be troubled, seems to me both reasonable and logical.

I tend to categorize patients into the following broad outline: (1) people who have problems; (2) people who are problems; (3) people who have problems and are problems or vice versa. Most of us like to work with a patient who has a problem. A problem is more definitive, less trouble, and more likely to have a beginning and an end. Unfortunately, most patients are people who have problems and are problems or vice versa. These people are more complicated, more taxing, more challenging, and in the long run more rewarding. The group two people, the people who are problems, are, in the present state of our knowledge, more difficult, more complex, and for the most part are beyond my training and competence. However, it is my responsibility to recognize these people, to refer them for psychiatric care or to arrange for some disposition which will permit them to live in the world with the least amount of disturbance to themselves and to others. Therefore, I feel it is my duty not only to diagnose the problem that presents itself as a patient, i.e., heart disease, liver disease, diabetes, etc., as it is to diagnose the patient who presents himself as a problem, i.e., conversion hysteria, hyperventilation syndrome, acute anxiety reaction with somatized complaints, alcoholic cirrhosis, etc.

So much for myself and so much for the patient. What else? For my part I find it necessary and profitable to read . . . to read about psychologic concepts, psychiatry theories and methods, books as well as journals, and in addition to read about man as seen by the non-medical person, for instance, the anthropologist; he has a lot to tell us about the development of man, his cultures, and the nature of man. In addition, I read the basic journals and texts of my field.

At last we come to treatment. I think it is a mistake to make something special of emotional problems. To begin with, I object to and I reiterate that I am not able to accept the dichotomy of mind and body. To me, symptoms and signs are language and they represent the expression of the state of the organism. In medicine we are so oriented to pathology that we forget that there are symptoms and signs of health. We tend to dismiss the healthy person as one who is lacking in pathologic symptoms or signs. However, we are neither trained nor appreciative of the symptoms and signs of health and frequently we tell a patient disappointedly, "I do not find anything wrong." Maybe we should tell him what we find right.

I believe that the patient has a personality structure or anatomy which is partly genetic and partly developmental, just like the rest of the body. For that reason, I want to know which members of his family he is like, whom does he feel like, and what are the characteristics of that person. I have people tell me, "I am like my mother, I feel like her, and I do not want to be like her." I believe that they are genetically like the mother and that we may be able to alter the responses if we know something about the mother and how she got that way . . . is she like the grandfather? I also believe that people behave in patterns and that the patterns are largely learned and that they repeat themselves like a conditioned reflex. Therefore, in the personality we find the reflex arc, i.e., the receptor organ, the mediating pathway or afferent nerve, the integrative or interpretative structure, the brain, again the mediating pathway or efferent nerve, and the reactor organ. I believe that this reflex arc can also be genetically conditioned to a certain extent and that there are patterns of reaction characteristic of races, nationalities, and families. In addition, there are the conditioning processes of life and living. If you are of the Freudian school, then you believe that the basic conditioning of the organism occurs in the family in the first six years of life. I believe this is correct and I can live comfortably with this concept as the basic premise on which to approach people and to try to understand them. I also believe that in this complex and marvelous organism something can go wrong besides conditioning and reaction. A collision with a noxious stimulus whether it be a bacterium or a fire truck, or over-stimulation, whether it be the TV or propaganda, or understimulation, whether it be deprivation or isolation, can disorder the organism. Internal derangements may also occur, such as endocrine imbalances or the collagen disorders.

Therefore, when the patient presents himself in a disordered state, this is an opportunity to explore and to understand as much about this disorder as is necessary to restore him to a functioning state of health or to assist him to adjust to his limitations. Frequently, it is the physician's own prejudices or sense of inadequacy that prevents him from asking the patient point blank, "Well, do you think this is a nervous condition?" In my own experience the patient is relieved that you have asked the question and generally there follows a flood of feeling and information. In my mind, a nervous condition is no different than a stomach condition and it is just as deserving of definition. I believe a gastric ulcer can be an angry ulcer and if we stop at the diagnosis of "gastric ulcer" and do not diagnose the anger, then our therapeutic horizons are limited because the diagnosis is incomplete.

Finally, to understand is not enough. Frequently, it is necessary to help the patient to take corrective action. If one has a deeply ingrained pattern of reaction which is inappropriate to the present and which interferes with his desired way of life, then the patient has to be retrained as to what is appropriate to the present, he must practice it, and he must reestablish new behavior patterns. In the neurotic person with insight, desire, and a grasp of reality, then I think much can be done to help this person. In the person who has not and will not develop insight, or who has no desire, or who distorts reality such as the psychotic, this person is beyond my reach and I must either refer him or turn him away. I do not think it is desirable or sound to try to put everything straight in a person's life. I believe that the best that can be done in my type of practice is to set the plan of therapy, to outline what needs to be done by the patient to get well, and to support him through the healing process with interest, advice, and medication where indicated.

Why do I chose to work with emotional problems? because

I believe they are no different than any other disorder of man and that they may merely be incipient symptoms of impending signs. Where does the peptic ulcer begin . . . in the cradle or at the table? How do I select the patients I will so treat? I doubt that I really select the patient; I believe he selects me to treat him. However, the patient must interest me, I must feel I understand his problem, and I must have the time in my schedule to undertake his case. Whom do I turn away? The ones beyond my training, the disinterested, the nonpsychologically oriented, the silly, the unreachable . . . and then, of course, there are some others.

REFERENCE

1. Asher, R.: A case of health. *Brit. M. J., i*:393, 1958.

PREPARING THE PATIENT FOR PSYCHIATRY

ZIGMOND M. LEBENSOHN, M.D.

THE WAY IN which a patient is referred to a psychiatrist by his physician is so vitally important that sometimes it means the difference between failure and success in treatment; between a long, slow treatment process and a rapid recovery; between an indignant patient and a grateful patient.

I do not think it is sufficiently recognized that the general practitioner is in a highly strategic position to tell his patient honestly and truthfully what to expect from psychiatry, and thus do a great service both to his patient and to the treating psychiatrist. On the other hand, even the best trained and most conscientious physician may unwittingly do or say something which may seriously delay psychiatric treatment or make it altogether impossible. Sometimes these errors are caused by the physician's uneasy feelings about psychiatry itself, which he unconsciously transmits to the patient. At other times, these errors are caused by fear, embarrassment or lack of knowledge on the part of the general practitioner when he deals with psychiatric matters. It is in an effort to allay these fears and embarrassments that this paper is being presented.

LICE AND PSYCHIATRY

I want to begin by telling a story. It is a true story and one which illustrates some of the pitfalls encountered in getting a patient to a psychiatrist. This will be followed by specific suggestions calculated to avoid these pitfalls.

A few years ago I received a call one morning from a successful young doctor who has a large general practice. I was with a patient at the time and was unable to speak but I returned the

10

call at my earliest opportunity. On reaching him, he expressed great relief. "Dr. Lebensohn, I'm so glad you called me back so promptly. I want to talk about a patient I'm sending you. Have you seen him yet?"

"No, I don't believe he's made an appointment."

"Good!" he replied; "You see, I gave him a slip with your name and address and told him to go right to your office."

There was a long pause and then I said, "I am very sorry but I don't think I will be able to see him today. If the matter is really urgent, I will try to make time for him as soon as I possibly can or try to get someone else to see him. What's the problem?" I asked.

"Here is the situation," he replied, "And this is why I wanted to call you before you saw the man. His name is Mr. Smith and he is a taxi driver. He came to my office complaining about body lice which were causing him to itch all over. He told me he had used several preparations suggested by friends and druggists but got no relief and the situation was driving him frantic. I was too busy to examine him but I gave him a lotion to apply locally and told him to come back in three or four days. He was back the following day. He said the lotion helped for a while but then the itching returned worse than ever. This time, I sent him into the examining room and had the nurse go over him with a bright light.. She couldn't find anything at all. I assumed the lice had disappeared even though the itching had remained, so I gave him another preparation with complete directions, and told him to return in about three days.

"He was back the following day, this time complaining that it was much worse. He seemed to be really bothered this time so I took him into the examining room and went over him myself with a fine-tooth comb. I was then convinced that he did not have lice then or at any time in the past. I told him I thought the lice were only in his mind and suggested he see a psychiatrist.

"Then he really got upset and he said, 'I was afraid you were going to say something like that. I had another doctor once who told me that, but I thought you would be different. I always thought a lot of you, Doctor, so don't give me a lot of that stuff! I know what I've got even though you can't find them.'"

The doctor continued, "Then I was more convinced than ever that he needed a psychiatrist so I told him, 'O.K., here is what I want you to do. I want you to see this doctor, Dr. Lebensohn. He is a specialist, a specialist in lice. He has a special microscope and he may be able to see these lice where I can't.' "

"So that is why I gave him your name and that is why I wanted to give you the background story before you see him, so you would know what to do."

Well, the story of this poor taxi driver is serious enough, but even more important are the lessons it teaches. Let us see now what actually happened. The taxi driver arrived in my office without an appointment, as instructed, noticed that the waiting room and office did not seem to go along with a "lice specialist" and, after introducing himself, he asked my secretary what kind of a doctor I was. She, of course, told him I was a psychiatrist, whereupon his face took on an expression of sour disgust as he said, "So that's the game!" turned on his heel and walked out.

One can hardly blame this patient for behaving in this way after being tricked into seeing a psychiatrist, even though his doctor had the very best of intentions. As a result of this well-meaning but unwise ruse, the patient was now more distrustful than ever of all physicians and became much more difficult to treat.

LESSONS TO BE LEARNED

Let us go back over the story, study the various errors, and see what we can learn. First, is the question of the referring doctor calling the psychiatrist before the patient comes in. At times, this may be very helpful but it is not always needed and is occasionally unnecessary. It depends to a large extent on how it is done. It is best to ask the patient what his wishes are. Sometimes a patient would prefer to see the psychiatrist without the benefit of a report which precedes him, a report which he fears may prejudice the psychiatrist. Often it may be necessary for the referring physician to call in order to obtain an appointment, but it is best to inform the patient.

Except for emergencies, most psychiatrists do not accept phone calls during the treatment hour, for obvious reasons.

Breaking into a therapeutic session may be like interrupting a surgeon in the middle of an operation. If a message is left, however, the psychiatrist will return the call at his first free moment. Sometimes it is a good idea to make the appointment with a secretary and to write a short note to the psychiatrist, giving the central facts and the reason for the referral. It is sometimes helpful to give the patient a copy of this note so that he knows exactly what has been said about him.

On the matter of getting an appointment, a frequent and important complaint in recent years, voiced by many of my good friends in general practice, runs somewhat as follows: "Here I work up a patient to the point where he or she will accept psychiatric treatment. Then I call up your office and find you aren't taking any new patients for one or two months. What is a man to do?"

This is a serious problem and the only way to solve it is to give the general practitioner a greater familiarity with the nature of the psychiatrist's work so that he can pass this on to his patient as part of the working-up or referral process. Due to the time-consuming nature of psychiatric practice, the number of patients any one psychiatrist can treat is necessarily limited. One psychiatrist can rarely see more than seven or eight patients in his office in one day, each interview lasting from thirty minutes to one-and-a-half hours. If he is conscientious, he knows that overloading his schedule results in fatigue and inferior work. Therefore, if you respect him as a psychiatrist, it is also important to respect his decisions regarding his ability to see a patient.

If he is not able to see a patient immediately and you think the patient can wait, it is helpful to explain this to the patient and advise him to do so. After all, the patient has probably had his difficulty for many months, and sometimes for years. On the other hand, if it is something which is more urgent, send him to another psychiatrist who has free time or ask your psychiatric colleague for other names. Ordinarily, a psychiatrist's schedule is made up some weeks in advance and he can usually tell you when he will have an opening. It is important to emphasize that it is almost impossible for the psychiatrist to do anything helpful for the new patient who is squeezed in between appointments.

It takes a full hour, and sometimes three or four, in order to find out what the problem is really about. Hence, it would have been of no help at all to see such a complicated case as the taxi driver for only a few minutes. This would only have antagonized him further. There is no substitute for time in the handling of delicate psychiatric cases.

CONSULTATION VERSUS TREATMENT

We come now to the subject of the one-time consultant versus the treatment referral. This problem is somewhat unique in psychiatry. If a psychiatrist sees a patient in consultation and recommends prolonged psychotherapy which *he* has the time to give, all goes well. If, however, he recommends treatment but has no time himself to see the patient for further therapy, the patient often feels cheated. The first consultation may have sold the patient not only on psychiatry, but also on that particular psychiatrist. Even if the patient is referred elsewhere, he feels that he has been unfairly treated, and so he has, unless it had been made abundantly clear to him by the referring physician and by the psychiatrist that the arrangement was to be for one consultation only.

Psychotherapy is such a highly personal matter that it is often advisable for both the psychiatrist and the patient to begin on a trial basis for three or four interviews without making any long-range commitments. If the psychiatrist does not feel that he is the right person for the task at hand, it is his duty to so inform the patient and help him make whatever other arrangements are necessary. Of course, it is the patient's privilege to withdraw from therapy at any time. It is important, however, for more physicians and their patients awaiting psychotherapy to know more about the psychiatrist and the way he works. Actually, his ways are not so unique or bizarre or unusual. His ways are dictated to a large degree by the exigencies of time but, to an even greater degree, by his special respect for the interpersonal aspects of the psychiatrist-patient relationship; and paying attention to the subtleties of the doctor-patient relationship is vital to all fields of medical practice.

THE MEDICAL WORKUP

We come now to the importance of the complete medical workup before making the psychiatric referral. There is nothing more dangerous, in my estimation, than the premature psychiatric referral with an inadequate medical workup. This holds not only for psychiatric but for all other specialty referrals as well. Had the taxi driver in our story been given a careful examination on his first visit, perhaps our story would have had a happier ending. By prescribing treatment for a condition which was not actually established, the doctor unwittingly reinforced the patient's delusions. When he finally examined the patient and found that he had never had any lice, he was placed in the embarrassing position of having to reverse himself. It was perhaps this very embarrassment which made the doctor reverse himself once again and participate in the patient's delusions by suggesting treatment for a condition which did not exist.

THE CRUCIAL IMPORTANCE OF HONESTY

In psychiatric referrals, I wish to emphasize (at the risk of coining a phrase) that "honesty is the best policy." There is no exception to this rule in referring a patient to a psychiatrist. Since honesty is important in all human relationships, it is all the more important in dealing with the psychiatric patient who has usually suffered from dishonest handling in the past and is particularly sensitive to untruths.

All deviations from the truth, no matter how innocent or well-meaning, invariably lead to disaster for all three—the doctor, the psychiatrist and, worst of all, for the patient. Place yourself in the patient's place. Wouldn't you want to know the truth, even if you chose not to accept the doctor's recommendations? In our story of the "lice specialist" it would have been far better had the doctor stuck to his guns. After discovering his first error, he should have told the patient that he was recommending psychiatric treatment. Even if it meant the loss of a patient, it would have been worthwhile for, ultimately, enough physicians would have arrived at the same conclusion to have made some impression on the patient.

Despite the progress that has been made in recent years, the word "psychiatrist" in some quarters is still considered not quite respectable. For this reason, there remain many diehards who make use of various substitutes, euphemisms and supposedly less shocking but inaccurate terms, such as "neurologist," "nerve specialist," "nerve doctor," and so on. If the problem is psychiatric and the patient is being referred to a psychiatrist, the doctor should say so. If the patient is deceitfully referred to any competent psychiatrist, he will learn his true identity in short order, and his confidence in the referring physician will be shaken. From experience, I find that much of the anxiety on this matter stems from the doctor himself and not from the patient.

Another temptation to which the family physician sometimes succumbs is well illustrated when he presents the following problem to the psychiatrist: "Now Doctor," he will say, "I have a patient who needs your help badly but she hits the ceiling when I mention the word 'psychiatrist.' Couldn't I simply tell her you are just a diagnostician or something, and let it go at that? Or better still, couldn't you just come to the house as a friend of the family? Or perhaps make a house call on her husband? I would be glad to arrange it for you."

Of course, yielding to any such deception is sanctioning the worst sort of medical practice. Under no circumstances should a psychiatrist ever be asked or permit himself to see a patient in any role other than his true one. In addition to being unethical, ineffective and actually harmful, such a ruse may get physicians into serious legal difficulties. Some years ago, a high ranking Army officer was anxious to have his very paranoid sister hospitalized before he left for an overseas assignment. She had been mentally ill for many years and had seen a psychiatrist once but had refused to return to his office for the second examination which was necessary for commitment purposes. The brother finally prevailed on two psychiatrists to join him in the cocktail lounge of a large hotel, where, by prearrangement, he was to meet his sister. The sister arrived and was quite shocked to find not only her brother but also two psychiatrists who spoke to her briefly and then filled out the necessary commitment papers.

Needless to say, the courts took a very dim view of the whole matter and, although the patient was very much in need of treatment, she was released by order of the court and the doctors were severely reprimanded.

TIMING THE REFERRAL

So far, I have confined my remarks to the "how" of referring a patient who needs psychiatric treatment. The question of "when" is sometimes more difficult to answer. It has been the hope of all enlightened psychiatrists to equip more and more of their medical colleagues with the essentials of psychiatry, so that they would be able to handle all but the most demanding psychiatric problems. In this connection, I would like to refer you to one of the most helpful books ever written on this subject. It is called *Psychotherapy in Medical Practice*, by Maurice Levine (1). It is not only one of best books written for physicians but also an excellent source for students interested in psychiatry.

It will never be possible, nor is it desirable, to send every patient with emotional difficulty to a psychiatrist. First of all, there are not enough psychiatrists to go around. Secondly, most of the milder emotional problems can be very successfully handled by the physician in general practice who has an interest and feeling for such matters. In general, there has been a tendency in recent years to refer the patient to the psychiatrist a bit prematurely sometimes, as in the case just cited, before the medical workup is completed.

Often the physician underestimates his own ability to manage the numerous emotional and psychiatric problems seen in the course of his practice. It rarely does any harm and it is most often of great help for the physician to continue to give the patient support and reassurance while waiting to see how the process is going. It is also wise to continue seeing the patient until he is accepted for treatment by a psychiatrist. Not every heart case needs to be seen by a cardiologist, nor does every emotional disorder need to be seen by a psychiatrist. In each instance, the knowledge of general cardiology and general psychiatry equips the general practitioner to treat many of these problems himself.

Obviously, the best time to refer the patient to a psychiatrist is at that moment when the physician has satisfied himself that he is no longer being helpful to the patient and that specialized techniques are needed. Sometimes a patient will anticipate his physician and suggest going to a psychiatrist himself, and sometimes even this may be premature. If so, the patient should be so informed.

INDICATIONS FOR REFERRAL

In most instances, the indications for psychiatric referral are quite clear. If any of the following symptoms are present, a psychiatrist is probably needed.

1. The persistence of incapacitating psychoneurotic symptoms, such as phobias, anxieties, obsessions or hysterical manifestations.

2. The persistence of psychogenic sexual problems.

3. The presence of psychotic symptoms, such as active hallucinations or delusions.

4. Sudden changes of personality or judgment.

5. Exaggerated swings of mood and motor activity.

6. The development of retardation, depression, and preoccupation with self-destructive thoughts. Sometimes a suicidal gesture which precipitates hospitalization by the family physician as an emergency measure may serve a useful purpose by bringing psychiatric help to a long-standing and reluctant patient.

WHICH PSYCHIATRIST

It is very helpful for the family physician to acquaint himself with the psychiatric facilities in his area. The best information is to be obtained from one of his psychiatric colleagues who will be glad to inform him on this score. In certain metropolitan areas where there are large numbers of psychiatrists, it is well to recognize that in psychiatry, just as in medicine or surgery, there are many different schools of thought and many sub-specialties within the specialty. For example, there are some psychiatrists who are specially qualified and trained in long-term psychotherapy or psychoanalysis; some who are equipped to administer the various forms of shock therapy; some who are primarily interested in psychopharmacology; others who limit their practice to office patients and do not have a hospital practice; and still others who limit their practice to those conditions which respond to intensive, brief psychotherapy. It is best to become acquainted with a well-rounded psychiatrist who is well trained in all the accepted techniques of therapy and rely pretty much on his judgment.

In this connection, it is unwise to tell your patient that he is being referred to a psychiatrist for the sole purpose of any *one* specific type of therapy such as electroshock therapy or psychoanalysis. The selection of the most effective treatment modality is often a difficult and time consuming task even for the psychiatrist. If the consulting psychiatrist should decide against recommending the specific treatment mentioned by the referring doctor, the patient is understandably bewildered. In the field of neurosurgery for example, it is not the custom for the referring physician to tell the patient that he is being sent to the surgeon for a suboccipital craniotomy. Of course not. The patient is simply told that he is being sent to another specialist for examination, diagnosis and recommendations for treatment. The same excellent principles should apply to a psychiatric referral.

IT PAYS TO BE SPECIFIC

Avoid vagueness in making psychiatric referrals. Vagueness on the part of the physician only leads to increased anxiety on the part of the patient. He is likely to think—"I wonder why Dr. Smith is referring me to a psychiatrist. Does he think I'm insane or something?" It is far better to be highly specific. Select a specific symptom as the reason for your referral. For example, you may tell your anxious patient something like this: "Your difficulty in speaking in public hasn't responded to medication. I think it would be helpful for you to see Dr. So and So, a psychiatrist, who is skilled in these matters." By focusing on a specific problem the anxious patient can more readily understand and accept the need for psychiatric consultation.

OVERSELLING

A frequent source of difficulty is the well-meaning physician who, in his attempt to get the patient to a psychiatrist, oversells psychiatry. By his efforts to allay the patient's anxieties, he may tend to minimize the difficulty or imply that, if he sees a psychiatrist, he will be completely cured in a few sessions. As you know, it is very difficult to estimate the amount of time required to treat any given condition, and it is best to suggest to the patient that most psychotherapy extends over a substantial period of time and rapid changes are the exception rather than the rule.

It is also unwise to oversell any particular psychiatrist for, should that psychiatrist be unavailable, the patient may have difficulty in transferring his confidence to another man, a second-best, so to speak.

The patient who has never consulted a psychiatrist is often quite concerned about what to expect from his first interview. A few words of reassurance from the family physician go a long way in allaying this anxiety.

The patient may also be concerned about the expense of psychiatric therapy and it is probably helpful to give the patient some idea of the prevailing fees in his community. If there is a serious economic problem, a special arrangement may sometimes be made with the psychiatrist or a psychiatric clinic utilized.

In general, the more a patient knows about what to expect from his first interview, the better it is.

SUMMARY

In summary, I should like to suggest the following ten points to aid the physican in referring a patient to a psychiatrist.

1. Always do a careful medical workup, even in the presence of obvious psychiatric illness.

2. Time the referral. Take enough time to establish a good working relationship with the patient before referring him to a psychiatrist. When you have done that, it becomes a meaningful measure and not a way of getting rid of a patient.

3. Never underestimate the ability of the sincere family physician to help the emotionally ill patient.

4. Be sure a psychiatrist is needed.

5. Be completely honest with your patient and with yourself. Tell him for what specific symptoms you are calling in a psychiatrist.

6. Avoid displaying needless anxiety or a sense of rush. Remember that there is nothing more contagious than fear.

7. Acquaint yourself with the psychiatrist and the psychiatric facilities in your area.

8. If you communicate with a psychiatrist before hand, inform the patient and tell him what you have said.

9. Don't oversell psychiatry or any particular psychiatrist, or any particular form of psychiatric therapy.

10. Tell the patient as much as you can about what he may reasonably expect from psychiatry.

REFERENCES

1. Levine, Maurice: *Psychotherapy in Medical Practice.* New York, Macmillan, 1942.

THE PHYSICIAN AND THE "CROCK"

ALVIN COHEN, M.D.

A NEW PATIENT came into my office and immediately began to talk about the pain in her back and how it had "nearly killed" her to just stand up and walk in from the waiting room. She directed her first remarks of pain to me and then did not notice me again. She went into intricate detail of the pain in her back and how sitting in various positions gave her pains in other parts of her body. She talked of her upper and lower extremities, discussing every joint. She went into a discussion of her teeth alignment and complexion. She spoke of various minute blemishes of her skin and talked of her G. I. Tract and other organ systems. She was like an artist as she painted a description of her body which was the most all consuming thing in her life. She had such love for her body that in a way she sounded like a person talking about a lover. Not only did she revel in talking about it herself, but she also assumed the examiner was equally enthralled. As she talked there was no question that this was all precious to her. This was her sole interest and she was sharing it with the examiner. If at any time during this recitation I had interrupted or interfered with the outpouring of material, this would have indicated to her a lack of interest and concern. She needed permission to continue and yet the more she ventilated the more steam she built up. She did not pause long enough for the examiner to make any comments and the same "organ recitation" was repeated at several successive visits. After a number of such visits, doctors often refer to this type of patient as an old "crock."

If we look up this word we find this slang diagnosis does not appear in the medical dictionary or Standard Nomenclature. It has no definition, being more a subjective term than an objective one. It is a doctor's diagnostic term having no meaning to patients. Included in the physician's concept of crock are patients who are overtalkative, chronic complainers, and those whose demonstrable organic pathology does not account for the symptoms. The patient might have major, minimal, or no organic pathology. Many different somatic and emotional illnesses fit the diagnosis, and the term applies to all types of psychiatric disturbances and in many different situations. The concept of hypochondriasis is as close as we can get to the theoretical counterpart of the term.

The hypochondriac utilizes his body to express conflict. Typically, the conflict is anger. These patients are angry; the doctors get angry; the word *crock* was coined in anger. We might speculate on the unknown origin of the medical use of the term. Crock or crockery is pottery. These patients are referred to by a word which might have evolved in medical language from pottery which is very fragile and easy to crack. It is interesting that even though these patients are referred to in such a derogatory manner, the term that is selected is one that implies fragility. It has been suggested that we call this a study of "psychoceramic psychiatry."

Many of these patients have the potential for a real break with reality, and hypochondriasis may be the symptom that prevents it. Often if hypochondriacal defenses give way, a psychosis may emerge.

Although the hypochondriac is the most common type of patient to whom the term crock is applied, if his symptom complex happens to fit in with the doctor's need, this patient is not so classified. A peculiar psychodynamic principle evolves: a crock is not a crock until there is established a particular type of relationship with the doctor, and it does not basically have to do with the presence or absence of disease. He only becomes a crock if he fails to augment the doctor's special interest. For example, if you believe that just about everyone has amoebiasis and a hypochondriacal patient comes in, you will not hear all the "head" and other body symptoms, but when you hear the bowel symptoms, the more vague they are the more you will love them, and then this patient is not a crock. This often accounts for some of the obscure cases of "amoebiasis" which respond to specific treatment, although no positive bowel diagnosis can be made. While on the other hand, a diagnosis of crock may be made if a patient does have an obscure case of amoebiasis but happens to go to a doctor who loves arthritis. We see then, that if a physician is obsessively interested in bowel function, his patient's symptoms can be molded and shaped to fit some bowel syndrome and a patient learns to talk about the symptoms which he knows interest his doctor. If the doctor has some new image he wants to foist on his patient, then the patient will not be a crock. Interestingly enough, the term is used more often to describe clinic or charity patients than private patients. In either case, the doctor should make up his mind to find at least one interesting thing about the patient, for the diagnosis is not made until the doctor has failed.

There are all varieties of hypochondriasis; the illness referred to in this paper is not the iatrogenic disease. Doctors may fall in line with this hypochondriasis but they do not cause it. They do not create the disease.

The hypochondriac demonstrates a type of narcissism (self interest) in which his emotional life is invested in his body organs and findings. He has retreated into his body. The energy, emotion, or feeling which otherwise would have gone into projects, objects, goals, and involvement with people is instead attached to body processes.

Hypochondriacal defenses are strong. These patients are frustrated and may become depressed. They have invested the body with a degree of concern and interest that makes it the sole and central reason for living and preoccupation. They manifest a cathexis of the body and body processes which is a substitute for object relatedness. The body becomes a substitute for interpersonal relationships. If they do establish any interpersonal relationships, they will be the kind that are sucking, demanding, and pleading. These will be one-way relationships. These patients say, "love me, love my body." The price for the relationship is that you must listen to their complaints.. If you do not listen to the symptoms, they will have nothing to do with you. "If you love me, you have to accept my symptomatology and hear me out."

When does this start? When does it come into being? We see children with hypochondriasis but do not call them crocks. We do not see many cases presented where the beginning of the illness can be clearly located. The illness is seldom identified when it first starts. It is more of a retrospective diagnosis. Most often it is a disease of unattractive, middle-aged, and older people. Young, attractive individuals are not called crocks.

When we speak of a hypochondriac, we are speaking of an individual whose defect is his inability to relate to things outside of himself; he is demanding attention. His ego functioning is intact but the investment of objects and ego meaning is absent. The outside world of reality is still there but it is not a valid substance of life. It does not bring satisfaction.

This patient delegates his infantile needs in a way that is a projection which cannot possibly come true. Then he can readily complain because he has delegated his needs to the doctor who cannot possibly meet his demands.

We more often than not get "fed up" with the patient who has an incessant torrent of symptoms. Why do doctors get disgusted with this type of patient? We hear this derogatory term, crock, when we first go into the wards at medical schools. It is a term used for patients we do not like; in the wards a previous doctor who makes the diagnosis warns the next doctor about these people.

What really concerns us about these patients is that they are an insult to our image of ourselves as doctors. We are angry because the patient continues to complain. He should be easy to cure, so the doctor feels a frustration and an ineptitude which the patient rubs in. They offend by virtue of their self-contained world of interest in their bodies. They really act as if they do not need the doctor. This is one of the first things they communicate to the doctor. They do not come and bolster him up and act as if he is going to cure them. They do not come with a preformed projected image of the physician as the great healer. All their fantasies are projected on their own apparatus. They come telling you that no other doctor cured them and you are not going to either. Most doctors assume, expect, and almost require a projection of positive feeling from their patients. With other patients there is usually an immediate positive transference to the doctor.

These patients, however, come in with no real expectation of getting rid of symptoms and no desire to get rid of this absence of expectation. They come in because they want to tell you about their body symptoms. They want you to be interested, but they do not give the praise, compliments, or thank you that the doctor has learned to expect. On the contrary, they are angry, hostile patients who arouse the doctor's negative responses. Nevertheless, the visit to the doctor's office is of considerable importance to these patients. They do not have a lot of things to do and the visit to the doctor might be the major event of the week. They are doomed to disappointment when the doctor is uninterested in listening.

The doctor ordinarily has trouble eliciting interview material from routine patients. He has to guess; he has to ask questions; he has to give cues; he has to slant; he has to focus; he has to cull. The crock does not require your help. The crock will come in, take care of the interview, and know all there is to be known. He pours out everything he wants to say and does not allow the intrusion of the doctor's knowledge and training. He makes us feel unimportant, unnecessary, inadequate and incompetent.

On the surface the crock comes in pleading, complaining, and whining, but the clear implication on a deeper level is that he is coming in expecting that you can do nothing. This certainly adds to the hostility exchanged between patient and doctor. The patient expects the doctor to neglect him. He actually has learned through previous experience that the doctor is not going to cure him and anticipates that the doctor is not going to be interested enough.

The diagnosis of hypochondriasis is not made quickly by a physician. Often, by the time he makes it, the patient has already gone to another doctor. A lot of doctors are able to establish good working relationships with the hypochondriacal patient. They play along with the patient; they give him the latest samples; they request on the chart a routine "crock work-up"; they take x-rays and call in consultants. It is interesting how some physicians can handle these crocks. They focus on a routine of a particular theory with the patients, attempting to use this to rationalize the clinical picture. They go through a whole repertoire of theories, trying to make it as drawn out as possible. They may eventually outline a theory of nervousness and diminish the tensions with drugs and often can keep the patient functioning adequately by this procedure.

The hypochondriacal patients usually begin the first therapy session by going through a recital of symptoms. They might do this over and over for several visits but eventually will get into discussion of some personal and social behavior. Treatment usually continues week after week and a year later they will probably still be going through the ritual, but they will have better relationships and will be doing better. They gradually get more involved with people and things, but continue to use their hypochondriacal defense. If the doctor gets too bogged down in trying to remove their symptoms, they do not improve. Do not force them to admit they feel all right, if you can get them to act all right. Let them feel their symptoms; they will still make many improvements in other areas, but we have to get them to stop saying they feel too bad to go to work. We can permit them to say they feel terrible as long as they go to work and are getting socially rehabilitated. We do not have to win the battle of admission. Often we must accept the fact that the symptoms are there and supply a need. They may be keeping the patient from becoming psychotic. Let the patient complain as much as he wants, but when you get a chance, go into such other areas as why did you lose the last job and how are things going between you and your mother-in-law.

A number of doctors have been keeping the crock satisfied for years and are quite aware of their own irritation about this type of patient. They have a certain fixed procedure they go through annually—some sort of a complete check-up. This will often be real and meaningful to the patient and will encourage him to let go of his symptoms after a thorough annual work-up. But this physical examination and reassurance alone is not what keeps the patient going. It is really what happens parallel to this that is crucial.

The vital ingredient the doctor is offering in spite of his frustration is an acknowledgment that this is a person who needs help. This is where psychotherapy comes in. The doctor must somehow develop the knack of getting into areas of the patient's life that are unrelated to symptoms. Ten minutes a week over a period of a year or two could enable the patient to start talking about feelings of depression and loneliness. It is all right for the patient to think repeated x-rays and other laboratory tests are necessary and important if the doctor remains acutely aware that the intensity of his interest can be his best therapeutic tool.

If the doctor does not maintain a good therapeutic relationship, the patients migrate. If the doctor adds an element of psychotherapy to what is presumably a good working relationship, a lot more would be accomplished.

The conscience plays a role in hypochondriasis. These patients have a strong sense of unworthiness. Some doctors find out what it is in life the patient feels most guilty about and a good deal of success in some treatments is due to the doctor's punitive attitude which gratifies some of the patient's guilt. Involved in a hypochondriacal system is depreciation, guilt, and satisfaction in self-punishment along with some infantile applications. These patients have a strong sense of right and wrong and a frequent unconscious mechanism is an attempt to actually do something to try to provoke the doctor to punish them, because punishment makes them feel better, e.g., the child after he has stolen the cookies has to be punished.

The doctor who is able to do a little more than just tolerate these patients has the beginning of good psychotherapy. If he adds a step, he can increase his effectiveness in management. Some doctors say that old Miss So and So likes to come in every week and must be given ten minutes or so of time and because of her complaints, he has to give her some kind of test. This perennial testing and deferring can continue and often accomplish something, but actually the doctor can be so much more effective if he simply adds a bit of curiosity about the person. If all the patient has is her complaints and her canary that she feeds every day, talk about the canary and you will have to spend less time than you would otherwise. Find some phase in this person's life outside of herself which she finds important—find the area of object relatedness. Find something important to the patient that is not a symptom and build around it. Find some little element which has not been swept away because of a narcissistic retreat. Objects are wiped out in narcissism and energy is invested in the body, but look for and find the little islands of contact—some relatedness in the world. Then gently, quietly, and unobtrusively acknowledge these little islands, always reminding the patient that he knows they are there. As the island grows, pay a little more attention to it and let the patient know you are interested. Always be on the alert to listen for an island instead of a symptom. If a patient grows something in her garden, let her tell you about it because all the rest of the time she may talk about her bowels, enemas, pills, and dizziness. Listen for a vignette of daily activity instead of a complaint about the "pills you gave me did not work." Talk to her about her garden and flowers. Ask her questions. This may cause her to retreat within seconds and return to her complaints.

You must use your judgment as to how often and how many tests are necessary to keep a ravenous, hypochondriacal hunger satisfied. You can not make changes immediately or quickly and sometimes you can not change it at all. Do what is necessary to keep the patient in rapport. Learn to understand the irritating feeling they evoke in you and how to handle it. Hostility that is seen clearly can be handled better. The patient also has to be helped to comprehend his unconscious hostility. He has overwhelming resentment to the world and some will definitely flow in your direction. Help him to alleviate his guilt and he will feel better. As increasing numbers of cures are accomplished medically, patients demand more and more from the physician.

In affording the patient care, which is after all our prime purpose, we, by the use of the term crock, automatically condemn the patient and thereby condemn ourselves and our thinking processes. Calling a patient a crock clangs shut an iron door and says in essence that we are not going to let in any new thoughts. Although I have used the word crock extensively in this paper, the cornerstone of good therapy necessitates the abolition of the concept crock. These are sick people. Let us continue to explore various therapeutic approaches until we learn to cure them.

REFERENCE

1. Bender, David: Seven angry crocks. *Psychosomatics,* 5:225 (July), 1964.

DIAGNOSING PSYCHIATRIC DISORDER DURING
A GENERAL MEDICAL EXAMINATION

JACK R. EWALT, M.D.

M ENTAL DISORDER IS a positive finding, and one which should
be based on detection of symptoms of feeling, thinking, or behavior which are typical of psychiatric disturbance; a diagnosis
should not be made because no other logical or somatic cause
for the symptom can be discovered. Furthermore, physicians
should always bear in mind that patients may have physical and
psychiatric disorders simultaneously. The psychiatric disorder
may be independent of the physical disease, may contribute to its
cause, or may be a reaction to it. A schizophrenic patient may
develop bronchopneumonia or acute appendicitis; a patient with
hypertension or peptic ulcer may have psychoneurotic components
which contribute to the pathology or accentuate its severity; a
patient with coronary disease, Parkinsonism, or advanced malignancy may develop a depression in response to his sense of
loss of his invulnerability.

Detection of neuropsychiatric disorders will result from
interpretation of the general symptoms uncovered in an ordinary
history or medical examination, not from the routine mental
status exam used for more detailed classification. Most of us
think we interpret general histories and physical examinations
in a purely objective manner, but in fact we tend to see in patients
the symptoms or diseases of interest to us at the moment, and to
interpret symptoms or behavior in terms of our own interest,
experience, and knowledge. Patients are often quite cooperative
and anxious to please, and leading questions frequently get us
into difficulty. The best questions for eliciting a history are

when? how? where? why? and, now and then, a discreet *who?*

This discussion is based on two general assumptions: first, that the family physician ordinarily is the first person to see patients with incipient mental disease or with great personality stress that may lead to mental disease, and that the detection must be done concomitantly with the routine procedures of taking the history and doing the medical examination. Many of the early signs of psychiatric disorder are the same as those found in somatic disturbances—thus it is necessary for the physician to consider mental disease among possible interpretations of the symptoms presented by the patients. Any significant change in the habits, behavior, weight, work, recreation, or other life processes of an individual which cannot be better explained by external facts or somatic illness should be thought of as evidence of incipient mental disorder. Certain changes that will become apparent in the course of the general history, observation of the patient's behavior, and during the physical examination are particularly indicative of psychiatric disturbance.

Changes in Food Habits

Well-nourished patients who say that they cannot eat a bite or that they have such chronic indigestion that they are unable to savor their food are always suspect. Psychoneurotic patients frequently have a whole battery of complaints concerning food habits and digestion, but tend to be of normal or excess weight for persons of their age and stature. Closely related is the patient who complains of gas in the stomach, abdominal pain, and fullness of the bowels in the absence of any objective evidence of gall bladder disease, chronic constipation, etc. Such patients are often neurotic or suffering from depression. Depressive symptoms are frequently referred to the gastrointestinal tract.

Many people are, throughout their lives, subject to food fads of one sort or another, but patients who have been reasonably sensible and suddenly go on a health kick or become food faddists late in life or during middle age should be suspect. Such patients are often either becoming neurotic or developing fantasies about changes in the body configuration or ego limits. These latter symptoms suggest either an incipient paranoid schizophrenia or a depression with somatic equivalents. Patients with depression frequently stop eating, and the event is documented by the loss of weight which accompanies it. The differential here will be between a malignancy or metabolic disease causing the weight loss and explaining the presence of the depression. Thus, inquiry as to the amount of food ingested (family members may be asked to check it) will often be valuable as part of the differential. Moreover, talking with the patient further will frequently reveal anger, hostility, and statements of depressed affect which are part of every depression.

Many patients become almost compulsive in their eating habits. Such compulsive overeating is seen in people who are using food as a tranquilizer. Some patients react to anxiety and insecurity over severe stress by taking frequent meals and by snacking almost continually throughout the day. The anxiety is often accompanied by sensations of hunger, and the patient feels temporary relief with satiation, but in a short time he is again in need of some oral gratification. At times, compulsive overeating may be a manifestation of a more serious disorder, such as schizophrenia. Some patients with schizophrenia symbolize love objects (which they wish to incorporate or, at times, destroy) as food; thus eating represents a form of gratification, but one that is never quite complete—and the dose must be repeated. In certain instances patients may, in a rather weird reversal, eat a lot to protect themselves against all aggressive feelings directed toward some loved person or respected physician. For example, one of our patients was noted by the family to be gorging herself on ice cream or, at other times, on blintzes. Inquiry revealed that the patient was quite angry with her therapist, had feelings that she would like to destroy him by eating, and feared that she would lose control during the therapeutic sessions. Therefore, for about twenty-four hours prior to an appointment she would gorge herself on some object which she equated with the physician. For example, she would imagine that Dr. M was a cheese blintz and then, with the magic of schizophrenic thinking, decide that he was *in fact* a cheese blintz. She would then go to the local store, buy a huge quantity of blintzes, and gorge herself on them for hours before her appointment. By the time the appointment came around, she would be so thoroughly sick of blintzes that the doctor was safe from all her aggressive feelings and she was less anxious during the interview.

In short, sudden changes in weight or sudden changes in food habits should alert the physician to the possibility of an anxiety state, stress reaction, depression, or a more serious psychiatric disorder such as schizophrenia. This consideration also applies to patients who have for years been overeating in a rather compulsive manner and who, by some leger de main, go on a rigid diet, drastically reducing their food intake. Sometimes such patients become depressed; one then learns that the food has been their way of combating severe depressive symptoms, and that the removal of their "medication" results in a flowering of depression. The same thing also happens occasionally with an alcoholic who has been "cured" of his alcoholism; that is, he commits suicide because of the depression that he has been watering down with the alcohol until he received therapeutic attention (or succumbed to our therapeutic zeal).

Changes in Sleep Pattern

Increasing sleep is a common symptom appearing early in an organic state or in patients who are surreptitiously taking sedatives. At times, one sees patients who respond to severe external stress by withdrawing into sleep. I don't believe we thoroughly understand why some people combat excessive anxiety by going to sleep while others become more tense, restless, and sleepless. People who promptly fall asleep when they travel by plane may actually be doing so as a method of dealing with anxiety. The student who develops hypersomnolence during the stress of finals, although he was previously able to prowl all night, may be reacting similarly.

The amount of sleep required by human beings apparently varies according to individuals more than is generally assumed. Persons who have a life-long pattern of insomnia or sleeping only a few hours are operating normally for them. But sudden decrease in amount of sleep is a danger signal; persons who have ordinarily slept a given amount, say six to eight hours, who suddenly develop insomnia are probably showing some type of psychiatric disturbance, of which anxiety states are perhaps the most common. Simple situational anxiety (pending examinations, important speeches, income tax time, marital problems, etc.) is probably the most common cause of interruption of sleep in our culture. The problem usually entails difficulty in falling asleep while a patient mulls over his situation, but in some instances the patient will fall asleep quickly but awaken early in the morning. Early morning awakening is most often found in depressions but certainly is not uniform—all types of sleep disturbance are seen in depressions. On the other hand, it is rare that a person with a full-blown depression sleeps well and does not show some decrease in sleep or disruption of normal sleep pattern. One finds broken sleep in organic states, and if the overwrought manic sleeps at all it will be in short catnaps.

Changes in Sexual Habits

Perhaps the most common detectable change in sex habits is a failure of potency in males too young to expect the usual physiologic decline. Females may also show a decreasing interest or ability for orgasm, but are more apt to manifest their disturbance via complaints of interruption or disturbance in the menstrual cycle. Anxiety and depression are the most common causes for disturbances in sex function in persons who have previously had a reasonably mature or adult pattern of sexual activity. Patients who have had lifelong sexual problems are usually neurotic or suffering from some type of sexual deviation; they present a different problem but one in which the sexual difficulty is apt to be the presenting symptom if it is mentioned at all. Phrased differently, persons with a habitual impotency, sexual deviation, or frigidity will come complaining of this symptom specifically or, if they come complaining of a somatic disorder may fail to mention this symptom. On the other hand, the person who comes with general complaints who has previously been sexually well adjusted will often have neurotic or depressive symptoms manifested somatically by disruption of his previously normal sexual adjustment, and once you have his confidence the patient will usually complain of it. As patients age there may or may not be a decline in frequency of intercourse in well adjusted couples; this seems to be a widely varying pattern and seems to be one of incentive and individual variation rather than one of specifically psychiatric disturbance.

Changes in Behavior

Patients with a previously reliable, conscientious work pattern may suddenly begin to goof off, quit jobs, and move from one to another. This may be due to undetected alcoholism. Quite often, however, these symptoms suggest an early stage of depression. Patients who have previously been satisfied with the job may decide that the job is no good, repressed anger against the boss may become explicit, and they move on.

A second kind of disturbance of work pattern appears in patients who become paranoid and begin to experience friction with their employees, fellow workers, or superiors. Paranoid delusions, irritations, etc. may result in rather marked disturbances in work pattern, such as constant job shifting, and usually there is some decrease in responsibility associated with successive jobs. On occasion patients who have worked very well develop a depression following promotion. Loss of the old job and the support and security it gave them, sudden exposure to increased responsibility, and emergence of a sense of guilt over maneuvers performed in the service of achieving the promotion may produce a depression.

Patients who are anxious or suffering from some external stress such as ill health, the situation of a family member, or financial problems may become preoccupied and increase their absenteeism, sustain injuries, etc.

A symptom more apt to be elicited from the patient's family or friends than from the patient himself whose presence usually suggests the onset of serious pathology might be categorized as change in social behavior or interpersonal relationships. There are about as many of these as there are types of human behavior, and only a few can be discussed here.

One of the most outstanding is typified by the person who suddenly shows a change in his pattern of morality. The longtime deadbeat lecher who reforms all at once may be suffering from a depression or severe guilt feelings; and it is somewhat ironic that such a development is usually seen, from the standpoint of society, as an improvement, while actually it may be indicative of serious individual psychopathology. (Of course, there *are* occasional cases of genuine religious or ethical conversion and real change in habits.) However, what is more common in our society is that people of previously abstemious habits suddenly become "immoral" or behave in a socially disreputable fashion.

Psychiatric disturbance may be expressed in sexual behavior directed toward young children or unsuitable adults of the opposite sex or in some type of homosexual or exhibitionistic deviate sexual behavior. These latter changes may be the manifestations of an early manic episode, but are much more commonly caused by incipient organic disease of the brain. When the aforementioned symptoms are associated with increasing irritability, general emotional lability, and difficulty in memory (particularly of the retentive type) one should ascertain whether an organic disease of the brain is present which is not immediately obvious on neurological examination. Patients who are becoming paranoid, either from schizophrenic or organic changes, may become unduly jealous or may develop marked prejudices toward people of different religion, race, nationality, occupation, etc. The symptom is particularly significant if the prejudice is new, that is, if a person who was previously tolerant of differences among people suddenly develops intolerance for one or several groups. Such people frequently become quarrelsome. In some patients the first manifestation of jealousy, prejudice, irritability, or quarrelsomeness is associated with and accentuated by alcohol indulgence. Friends often notice that the patient's alcohol tolerance is lower, and that although previously he could drink like the proverbial gentleman, he now becomes irritable and out of control on two drinks or so.

Another type of person who is probably showing signs of an incipient psychiatric syndrome is the one who has involved himself in a long series of legal entanglements. While ordinary people may get involved in a series of litigations, in most of those in which pathology is the major motive the issues are of the nuisance type and are based on flimsy grounds. A similar type of behavior occurs in the person who begins to mismanage his financial affairs so that they are grossly confused in spite of an adequate income.

These latter two types of behavior can be seen at work in persons with paranoid coloring, and especially in persons with paranoid organic syndrome. Manics may also get into financial difficulties, but in such cases the problems usually include over-expansion of debts, unwise purchases, unwise contracts, etc. The quiet, reserved person who becomes noisy, talkative, quarrelsome, and overactive is probably showing early symptoms of a manic disorder or some type of organic disorder, especially one involving the frontal lobes.

Reasonably neat people who become slovenly, unkempt, and careless about their appearances are probably suffering from incipient organic disease. They are apt to appear with shirttail out, trousers not properly fastened, shoes untied, etc. While advanced schizophrenics show similar characteristics, a person in early stages of an illness who shows this type of symptom is more likely to be organic.

In general, one should suspect some type of mental pathology when a person begins to change in his behavior in a way inappropriate to a person of his education and profession and to the time and place in which the action occurs. For example, if I came to give this address in coveralls and with greasy hands my behavior would be suspect. If, on the other hand, you found me working on my sports car dressed as I am now (except during a roadside emergency) *that* would be inappropriate and you would be justified in wondering what was going on.

If any of the other changes mentioned above are encountered in the general history and physical of a routine medical examination, one then turns his attention to more accurate estimate of changes in the mental processes. The one most easily detected and most commonly complained about by patients is change in memory—forgetfulness, absentmindedness, and capricious memory warn of impending organic deteriorations of the mental processes.

Unusual elation, euphoria, or overactivity during the examination are indicative of early manic syndromes; blocking, depression, slow repetition are typical of severe depression, and will become apparent to the physician. Recurring thoughts of obsessive ideas seen in neurotic states, or sometimes in the early stages of schizophrenia, will also be noted during the ordinary history-taking. Estimates of defects in judgment are more difficult to accomplish during the initial examination, and some extra investigation, such as inquiries directed to family or business associates, may be necessary.

Early detection of mental illness, particularly those forms that may lead to impaired judgment and to business, financial, or personal problems obviously is important. An ordinary, careful history elicited by the family physician will reveal incipient psychiatric disorder if the patient's symptoms are seen as being possibly explained by neuropsychiatric disturbance. A patient who is fatigued, who has lost weight, and who complains of indigestion and loss of appetite may indeed have a malignancy of the stomach, but he may also have a depression; or he may have a depression without any overt gastric pathology. Once alerted to the possibility of a psychiatric explanation for the patient's symptoms, most physicians are competent to make a diagnosis that something is wrong and they can then, through further examination, elicit symptoms which confirm the diagnosis. Or they may prefer, at that point, to refer the patient to one of their psychiatric colleagues. The choice will depend on their personal wishes, skills, and experiences, and on the availability of a psychiatrist with whom they can work.

PANEL DISCUSSION

MODERATOR: JAMES A. KNIGHT, M.D.

PANELISTS: SORUM, EMORY, LEBENSOHN, COHEN AND EWALT

Dr. Knight:

IT IS A GENUINE pleasure to serve as moderator of this distinguished panel. The participants on this panel have spoken to you today and shared with you a rich abundance of material drawn from their clinical practice and research. They now welcome your questions and comments. Discussion is encouraged between panel members as well as between panel and audience.

Dr. Sorum:

Since for some reason you happened to look over at me, I wanted to make a point based on what Dr. Cohen has said. Someone was asking me about his paper on the crock, which I thought was so splendid. He discusses how many of these pepole have to be left with their symptoms. What they need is relief and a shift of support. They seem to need these symptoms as a certain type of defense. It is the way they have of orienting to the world and of clinging to reality. I thought this was a very good point. I once had a paranoid, though she didn't present herself as one, who was a nun wearing a habit. She kept asking why she had to wear this habit which she had to look at every time she looked one way or the other. This seemed reasonable at first, until I began to get into her case further. Then I felt strongly that if we took this habit away from her, she would develop a widespread, galloping paranoia. I told her this was one of the things that she just had to do and talked to her superiors about it. They agreed

40

that she had other incipient paranoid ideas. This is a good example of somebody we left with a "hypochondriacal" referential point in order to keep her from getting something worse. She was essentially a crock. She would talk for hours about how terrible this habit looked and yet, without it she would have decompensated.

Dr. Ewalt's remarks threw me into a panic state. I must explain that I had lost about a hundred pounds over a two year period. You talked about changes in personality in people who had lost weight, and I was sitting there getting quite frightened and very hungry.

Dr. Ewalt:

I still contend that people who overeat are doing it for a reason. Why you decided you could lose weight, whether you've taken up drinking or those cigars, is something I don't know.

Dr. Emory:

About that time I sent a patient to Dr. Sorum, and Dr. Sorum lost weight but the patient gained weight.

Dr. Sorum:

I know why it happened. I was doing hypnosis at that time and a patient was sent to see me. I weighed 330 pounds at the time she walked into the office. The patient sat down and started talking, then abruptly started to leave. I asked "Why are you leaving?" and she said, "Well I came here to get rid of my obesity, and look at you!" I think that must have been the reason.

Dr. Lebensohn:

While we are on the subject of food, I'd like to respond to Dr. Ewalt's paper. Before I do I would like to say that I was well impressed by all the papers this morning and this afternoon. They seemed to fit into each other without collusion or pre-arrangement. This speaks well for a unitary point of view on the part of the speakers. As a result, I hope that this symposium will be more enlightening than confusing to the audience.

To come back to Dr. Ewalt, I must take strenuous issue with

his disparaging remarks about blintzes. I consider them a great delicacy. I don't have several "attics full of them," but blintzes (derived from the Russian word "blini" meaning pancakes) are made like Crêpes Suzettes, wrapped around flavored cottage cheese and served hot. They are eaten with sour cream, sugar and cinnamon. I think the trouble is that Dr. Ewalt hasn't been subjected to the right kind of blintzes in the past. Furthermore, I'd like to add that any blintz is a good deal more tasty than any psychiatrist I know. Since attacking her psychiatrist was a problem in your patient's case, I think she was well advised to eat these blintzes.

Another point that Dr. Ewalt made deserves a good deal of emphasis, and that was the importance of getting reliable objective data from patients. When he talked about insomnia, we learned that some of these people actually sleep a great deal more than they report and that their complaint is more illusory than real. This reminded me of a case of ejaculatio praecox which was reported many years ago in the *International Journal of Psychoanalysis* by the late Dr. Bose, a psychoanalyst in Calcutta, India. He described a man who complained of ejaculatio praecox which was threatening his marriage. He was in treatment for some time when Dr. Bose finally suggested that he produce some objective data so that the doctor would have some idea as to what he really meant by the term "ejaculatio praecox." The patient then proceeded to time himself and reported that his average time, from the beginning of sexual intercourse to its culmination varied from thirty to forty-five minutes! Dr. Bose asked his patient how he could justify the complaint of premature ejaculation in light of such well documented sexual control. The patient replied "Well, I still have not been able to bring my wife to orgasm!" The case, needless to say, was finally resolved by treating the wife's sexual frigidity.

Audience:

I'd like to ask about the woman in her middle years with pelvic complaints that you treat, treat and treat and she has pelvic pain and tenderness and dyspareunia and finally, in desperation, she has surgery, and the pathologist gives you a clean report. You assume that you've made a mistake and you're gonna have another crock on your hands with adhesions as you mentioned, but she suddenly gets well. She has no further complaints. She's a happy woman. How would you explain this?

Dr. Cohen:

There are several possible explanations. I'll mention some. Actually, we must realize that any intervention with a surgical, medical or psychiatric procedure brings with it a multitude of possible reasons for results. We don't always know why results are good or why they are bad. We don't always know in what way we might have touched on some crucial, deep emotional need. We recognize that punishment of some type, inflicted on some types of patients often results in improvement. We know sometimes patients respond to suggestion. I remember in medical school when we sent some borderline literate people to get x-rays and they didn't know that this was just a test, they'd come back and say, "I feel better." Patients who received venipunctures sometimes didn't understand that they were just having a test made and would say that they felt better. I think the suggestive element of what happens in any therapeutic procedure is pretty powerful. I would also feel, though, that if we followed this type patient over a number of years the relapse rate would probably be pretty high. Many of the surgeons who do this type of procedure report that several years later there is another area of involvement, such as a depression or other organ symptoms and the patients need additional treatment. If this one shot deal works for a lifetime recovery, I think that's marvelous. Actually there are so many factors responsible for so-called cures it is hard to say why some patients improve and some do not. If a patient does well and stays well after surgery it means the need was met for that particular patient at that particular time. We can't generalize and say such surgery is good for all patients, all the time.

Audience:

You think that possibly there's something there that the pathologist can't find that we did cut out? Is it possible that she could have had a psychic trauma that coincidentally was removed about the time of her surgery and as a result of that there might not be a recurrence due to a psychic experience that had resolved itself in the course of events.

Dr. Sorum:

It's possible that her dependent needs were met by being sick and having something done for her. I saw a case last year of a girl that I knew was schizophrenic. She developed abdominal pain, and finally developed an acute pain in the right lower quadrant. She had a rising sedimentation rate. I thought that nothing was organically wrong. I discussed with the surgeon the possibility that surgery wouldn't help. The operation was performed, and there proved to be really nothing the matter, but she did feel much better. I asked her later why she felt better. She said, "Every day you came to see me. I could only come to see you once a week or so, but every day you came to see me. My mother came to see me. My friends came to see me. I had friends." Now the magic has worn off in this case. She has again decompensated. Along with her dependency she does seem to have a lot of hyperacidity and pain, so apparently there's no choice but to again perform the tests. I think they'll think twice about surgery this time, but she did have her needs met for a while. For a while she relaxed and had these memories to live on having been helped and reporting back to doctors and people showing active concern with her. I notice that she shows some symptomatic improvement when I let her talk at length about her diet. Unless her needs are met in some supportive way, she has a return of symptoms.

Dr. Lebensohn:

The doctor's question brings up an issue which is vitally important in both psychiatry and medicine. Perhaps what was done for that patient was just the right thing and was more effective than any kind of uncovering therapy. We don't really know. Simply because a person recovers or his symptoms subside following a certain procedure does not mean that he recovered *because* of that procedure. This is unscientific reasoning. We sometimes do not know, even in intensive psychotherapy, why people get well. Sometimes the reasons we suggest are not those which the patient considers important. When I was on the staff of St. Elizabeth's Hospital in the thirties I made a practice of asking patients about to be discharged the following questions: "What form of treatment caused your recovery?" This was before the era of shock treatments, tranquilizers and so on. You might expect they would say "The psychiatrist, the psychotherapy or the group therapy." Not at all. The psychiatrist came way down at the bottom of the list. Most of them replied "The hydrotherapy, the packs, the tubs." This was something tangible, something that meant something to them. Now we all know very well that it was the total experience, plus time, plus many other factors which went into their recovery, but the patients, themselves, were not able to articulate it. Therefore, from the scientific standpoint, we do not know why your patient got well without making a most careful investigation. We can't make that investigation because, by the very process of making that kind of an investigation we would run the risk of making this person sick again.

Dr. Emory:

There would be two things that would come to my mind in a situation like this. One would be—and this is a castration procedure—this lady may have had considerable problems relative to pregnancy or to sexual problems and this is a castration procedure and this may have relieved her of this problem but she may only show you the face of being well, of feeling well and wanting to be well, which may be really masking an incipient depression which may appear years later. I think many of these people who have these pelvic operations do develop depressions later on, or guilt feelings and depression.

The other thing that would come to my mind in situations like this is that people sometimes get sort of trapped with symptoms. They've lived through these behavioral patterns, these acts, long enough and they need a way out. An operation is a very acceptable procedure. There is a certain element of punishment that goes along with an operation and they're cleansed in this respect and this gives them a socially acceptable way to get out of the problem and the symptoms that they've carried so long.

Dr. Ewalt:

I certainly would agree with what's been said, particularly these latter remarks. There's one other thing I think should be mentioned and that is that the sample on which one bases such evidence and such statements quite often is a biased sample. This happens in psychiatry, too. We make the generalization that schizophrenics come from broken homes. This was fine until they started surveying communities and found there are more well people from broken homes than there are schizophrenics, and so forth. What happens is that your patients who are happy and contented with you tend to come back, but those who decided you did something rather bad may drift off to other places. I could quote some literature from twenty-five or thirty years ago about a surgeon who used to report the same thing. He must have taken out three barrels of ovaries, and he used to report a great many improvements regarding neurosis. On the other hand, I had the misfortune to be out at the University Hospital where all his "cures" came when his surgical cure wore off and there wasn't anything else to take out. So I think one has to be very wary of just accepting, on an impressionistic basis, our apparent results. This does not apply only to surgeons. It is true of psychiatrists, too, in their evaluations of drugs, psycho-analysis (I happen to be an analyst), dynamic psychotherapy, and all these other things. When you really put it onto a hard, valid sampling system, you find out a lot of these things we know just aren't so.

Dr. Cohen:

We find out, too, that no matter what procedure, technique or drug you use a certain number of people respond positively and a certain percentage do not.

Dr. Sorum:

Of course, I imagine if you did this surgery, it was done with a lot of support, encouragement, and a good relationship with the patient, too. This is going to help. If you are doing this thing with an air of, "Let's try this and see if it works," I think it's probably not going to work. At least the results for awhile depend a lot on the attitude with which the contact is made.

Audience:

We also have patients that will come in and will have the same symptom. I've seen this also in patients who had backache. You say, "Did you go back to see your doctor? Did you tell him you still had backache?" "No. I did one time and it made him feel bad." They support the doctor, sensing that he had some need in this, too, and went somewhere else and complained about it.

Dr. Sorum:

That's a good point, and I think it occurs frequently.

Dr. Emory:

It seems to me, in my own practice, that many of the women with multiple complaints actually are afraid of getting pregnant and giving them instruction in birth control or, perhaps as was done here, removing the uterus removes many of the symptoms that they have been describing previously. As you said, we don't know what happens years later.

Audience:

I would like to ask Dr. Ewalt about sleeping pills. Do you have any solution to the problem of many people who just have to have a sleeping pill at night before they go to bed? Should they be removed, if possible, because of the danger of addiction, or is this something that is significant to this person's well being?

Dr. Ewalt:

I don't think one can answer the question simply or categorically. In the first place, I believe that when a person starts on the sleeping pill kick you ought to try to find out why he needs these things, or *if* he needs them, and try to remove the cause. Now after a person becomes addicted, it's just cruelty to take it away abruptly. I think it's much harder, at that point, when he has developed not only a physiologic but also a mental dependence, to take them away entirely. I think it takes some very nimble-footed psychotherapy and support to get him off. I think any psychiatrist or other physician who reports that this is easier, that he has a high degree of positive results, is either not counting fairly or is lying, or just has had one or two lucky cases. Now occasionally you can get patients to convert. I haven't had a long series of these, but I had one lady who was taking Nembutal®. We worked on this a little bit and she remained dependent on Nembutal. She didn't have to take it any more, she just had to *have* it. It turned out that she was so afraid she wouldn't sleep she would take it. So I gradually persuaded her. I said, "Well listen, put the pill and a glass of water beside your bed. If you can't sleep, you can take it." She found she could cut the dose down, and finally she was using about twelve capsules a year. Every night she'd put the pill down, put the glass of water down on her bedside table, and go blissfully off to sleep. Next morning she'd put the capsule back. These capsules don't stand up very well, and she'd wear out about a dozen a year. She was still completely dependent on this procedure but she didn't have to take the pill—just needed it to be there so she could take it if she had to.

Dr. Sorum:

It acted as an amulet—somewhat like substituting with a ritual. There are people who report good results on hypnosis and conditioning for the same thing. Often when you teach the patient a lot of exercises to induce sleep or to relax, this does substitute the ritual, or at least for a time while it's being reinforced. There have been some good results with that. I've seen some who have began developing other symptoms. One of them joined the Unity Church. I thought she'd gotten off the pills well, but she finally told me that the church to which she went told her that it was sinful to take pills. It's a strong transference, not to me, but to the practitioner. This finally got her sleeping. As far as I know, it's still working. I'm glad.

Audience:

Since the nervous system only metabolizes carbohydrates, what effect does it have on the nervous system or do you believe this?

Dr. Sorum:

I don't know about that. I've had a number of patients who have come in with literature on the subject, saying they felt better from following its suggestions. There's a book out called *"Body, Mind and Sugar"* which claims much success, but beyond an awareness of the idea, I don't know enough to answer the question.

Dr. Emory:

There are types of hyperinsulinism. They are generally in the nature of a tumor of the pancreas. There is also some accompanying hyperplasia of the pancreas. But the every day run of obesity, in itself, I do think is not primarily based on hyper-insulinism and I don't believe that the appetite is primarily related to the pancreas. I don't know of any clinical laboratory process by which we can demonstrate a hyperinsulinism if we suspect it. There are sophisticated research methods for assaying insulin. Patients with hyperinsulinism are unusual cases and these generally are pancreatic tumors. Obesity isn't necessarily an accompaniment either.

Some people don't tolerate carbohydrates as well as others. They metabolize somewhat differently. I think that some people become practically addicted to carbohydrates and that there is a disturbance in metabolism somewhat related to diabetes. Many people tend to be obese if they eat high carbohydrate diets and frequently in dieting all I ask people to do is to reduce or cut out the white foods. They handle this restriction very well and they lose weight. Alcohol is one of the white foods, and it doesn't take but a little bit of alcohol, in many people to bring the weight right up, and alcohol is addicting.

A diabetic feels very much better when his sugar is around 110, 120 than he does when it's 80. He's extremely irritable when his blood sugar runs 80. There must be some relationship.

His tissues also adjust to a higher level. Some even feel better at 150 or 180, too. Some people are very hard to regulate. I think there are shifts in metabolism over a period of time in a diabetic, where they may have a tolerance to carbohydrates.

This is true in other fields. The hypertensive. If you bring them down too fast they feel bad and sometimes will stop the medication. The body adjusts to specific levels in many categories.

Audience:

Is it permissible to allow a crock to more or less dictate his treatment? I have in mind a patient who has numerous complaints and she'll come in and say, "My colitis is bothering me again." I know, from all we know medically and can find that she doesn't have coltiis, she has no recognizable symptoms or findings of colitis. I go along with it and I treat her for colitis. Her definition of colitis is a vague, uncomfortable feeling in the abdomen. Is it permissible to agree with them and go ahead and treat them and then wait until her next symptom comes up and treat it?

Dr. Cohen:

You're treating a patient in keeping with her diagnosis which you know is incorrect. But you have established good rapport with this patient and she is responding. If she has a need to have colitis and you understand this particular need, and can alleviate her symptoms with simple drug treatment and her "attacks" are infrequent, you are handling the patient adequately. You shouldn't let a patient dictate harmful treatment but if the request is harmless and helpful, use it. I think that's perfectly permissible.

After all, we're always really responding to the patients demands on us. We might say, "We are the boss," but in truth we often can only do what the patient wants or to express it more exactly we can only do what the patient will permit us to do. The patient calls the signals by accepting or rejecting our tests, drugs, advice, and other treatment. Sometimes what the patient wants is to have the doctor be angry at them. Sometimes he wants us to give him a certain test. Sometimes he does not want us to do a certain test. If you have good rapport and are getting symptom relief, that's a good relationship with the patient. Of course, you can't possibly permit a patient to dictate against medical judgment to the extent of inflicting serious harm by omission or commission.

Dr. Lebensohn:

I'd like to carry this on a bit further. I have been in practice long enough to see what happens to "crocks" of this type who, over the years, have trained one physician (after trying many) to do just what they have needed. Then this doctor dies, leaves town or retires. I have seen such people collapse because they have reached that point in life where they don't have quite the energy to train another doctor to their "way of life." This can become a very serious matter which merits our attention. It is also related to the previously mentioned tendency of doctors to ride a hobby. Dr. Cohen told us about the doctor who was interested in amoebae. Every patient he saw was a potential case of amebiasis because that was the one illness which deeply interested him. It reminds me of the story about the young doctor who was taking over the large country practice of a retiring physician who had been most successful. On meeting him for the first time he said "I understand that you've had a most remarkable success with patients." The old man, who was beginning to get a bit senile, fiddled with his vest pocket and finally pulled out a little white pill. "You see this pill, son?" "Yes, sir," the young doctor replied, "What is it?" The oldster answered, "Well I don't rightly know, but I give it to all my patients." "What does it do?" asked the young man. "Well, it gives them fits, and son, I'm just hell on fits!"

Audience:

Dr. Lebensohn, they tell us to be careful about a patient that starts talking about taking his life. You mentioned something about "Watch out for legal action and so forth." I'm kind of confused now. We are told to put the patient under the care of a psychiatrist. Supposing the patient that has tried to commit suicide refused psychiatric help?

Dr. Lebensohn:

If the patient refuses, and you have exhausted all the means at your disposal and the patient's family also refuses, I don't think you can do much more. From the legal standpoint you must operate within the framework of the laws governing the mentally ill in your jurisdiction. One may argue this point philosophically and say that a person has the right to take his own life and that he does have the right to refuse treatment. As physicians, we do not know *for certain* that this person is going to take his life. However, we can say on the basis of our training and experience that this person is depressed and the likelihood is great that some harm will occur. We can say all this to the proper authorities and we can urgently recommend treatment in a psychiatric hospital. If it is the judgment of the responsible physicians in the case that there is a real risk of suicide then the necessary legal steps should be taken to have that patient hospitalized even if it is against his will. You have a perfect right to do this, provided you operate strictly within the laws of your jurisdiction.

Dr. Ewalt:

There's one thing I'd like to say about this suicide business. It is a great problem, particularly if you run a hospital, as we do, where patients come in to the emergency room. Quite often a person who is depressed and thinking of committing suicide, and has made previous attempts, can make an agreement with you, which they usually keep, to talk to you about it, say the next day. You don't try to get them to guarantee that they won't commit suicide. I don't know that they can, so it's asking the impossible. Most of them can agree to postpone it, and you can talk to them about it.

I have, right now, lots of patients running around Boston who, if they called the hospital, would be told where I was. When the call came I would go out and take it. I wouldn't ask anyone, "Now promise not to commit suicide." What I would say is, "I'll be home Saturday afternoon. We'll talk about it then." That way they feel that you're interested in them, but you're not asking them to do the impossible. A lot of them can make the commitment from day to day, although they can't make the more or less permanent commitment to you.

Don't ask them to call you and then have them find that your secretary is not allowing them to get to you or that you're out on the golf course, because if they feel that they've lost you and you're not in, that's when they may make another attempt. So try always to be available if you said you would be. When I fly around in airplanes on these trips I tell them, "You won't be able to get me from this hour to this hour because I'll be on an airplane. But if you leave word at the place I'm going to I'll call you back as soon as I get there." They don't do this very much —probably once a month on trips like this I'll get a call from such a patient. The fact that they know they can reach me is what counts. Very often they'll check to see if they can, and that's the end of it.

Audience:

I was thinking of this officer's sister. Supposing she was a potential suicide and the psychiatrists had put her in a hospital for that reason to protect her?

Dr. Lebensohn:

First of all, the case in question was not depressed or suicidal; she was paranoid. Had she been depressed and was still depressed and suicidal at the time she appeared before the judge, the judge would not have ordered her release. He might have still reprimanded the doctors for the way they committed her since there was a much better way of doing that even in the District of Columbia. You can almost always persuade a police officer by saying "This person is going to commit suicide unless she is placed in custody." They can almost always be persuaded to take such patients into custody.

Curiously enough, many of you who are living in smaller communities have a much easier task in getting patients into a hospital than we have in the larger cities, where the rules are extremely strict. Woe unto those who deviate from them! They are often sued for malpractice before they have time to turn around.

Dr. Knight:

I could make a comment in that line. In this state, at least, if such a situation would arise it should be turned over to your parish coroner who has political immunity from prosecution for a false commitment, if he acts in good faith.

Audience:

Psychiatrists do differ, and as another psychiatrist I would like to differ with Dr. Cohen—not differ, but maybe emphasize that what's comfortable for one of us to practice may not be comfortable for another. We have our techniques and this would be applicable, I think, to the general practitioner. Dr. Cohen mentioned that he permits, or thinks that x-rays may be requested when a crock—he emphasized abolishment of that term—wants it, as long as the physician maintains his relationship. I think this may be comfortable for some general practitioners but I still adhere to the view that many have held. That is, that, when you do have a hypochondriachal patient, that it's important to give them a thorough physical evaluation, as thorough as thorough can be. But then stick to your guns when, a month later, they want another electrocardiogram, another chest xray, unless there are some most unusual circumstances, because I think back in the mind of the hypochondriacal patient in spite the physician stating, "Now I know there's nothing wrong, but just to further reassure you, I will do this exam. I assure you I know there's nothing wrong"—the hypochondriacal patient is telling himself that the doctor still has enough concern to once more listen to my heart, to once more request an x-ray. Therefore I believe that you have to show your own certainty by saying, "You've been thoroughly examined." What I do with hypochondriacal patients is often set up a schedule whereby I say,

"Now I want you to go back to your internist or general practitioner in six months," and when five months comes, I will remind them, "You're a month off from your *regular* examination." Now Dr. Cohen and I have talked about this point, so I'm not springing anything on him—we do differ. Again, it's a technique of the physician. This is what I've been hearing all morning and all afternoon that what's comfortable for one practitioner may not be comfortable for another, and vice versa.

Dr. Cohen:

I wouldn't argue with the idea that the doctor has to stand for something. He has to set a certain code of behavior for himself, he has to express himself with some degree of certainty, but I think what's therapeutic is the doctor's certainty, rather than whether you set a six-month interval for examinations, or whether you check the heart every visit. I think it's the doctor's attitude that is more important than the ritual. The patient should always have the feeling that "The doctor is interested in me. He's still communicating with me. He's still concerned about me." If an authoritarian approach should convey to the patient, "You don't care if I'm having a heart attack or not," this patient will leave you. It is what the patient interprets from our behavior that's important, not what we mean. I'm working on the assumption that you can't work with a patient unless he continues to be your patient. Keep your patients coming to you. That is a must. You have to. You may develop whatever procedures that work well in order to keep things going until you can blend in your psychotherapy. If the doctor feels most comfortable doing reexaminations of hypochondriacs at a rather fixed, semiannual time interval that is all right. But if other doctors feel more comfortable in being more flexible about it, that will not hurt treatment. I don't think the time interval or frequency of examinations is the important point. I think the doctor's attitude is the crucial point.

Audience:

I was going to say that hypochondriacal people do have heart attacks, as others do. This was exemplified in my practice not too long ago. This lady had been to see a physician and he had checked her thoroughly and three days later she called him to her home. He just thought she had another complaint. He put her in the hospital and didn't even take an electrocardiogram. So she discharged him promptly and secured another physician. She had had a coronary. So they do get sick.

Audience:

I want to direct a question to Dr. Emory. You talked this morning about these patients. Once you had seen them and decided they had a problem or they were a problem or a combination of both, you then decided whether you could help them or you couldn't help them or whether they were to go somewhere else. Tell me, diplomatically how do you get rid of them?

Dr. Emory:

It's not just a matter of getting rid of them. I can't treat everybody. Some people I can treat, and some I cannot. If I have a pateint who has a surgical problem, I tell him simply this is not in my field, I'm not competent to handle this, but I'll see that he gets into good hands or I'll give him the names of the surgeons, or who is his physician for this particular type of work. I don't think you have to make any difference whether this is a psychiatric referral or whether it's a surgical referral or any other kind of referral. There are some people who really aren't interested and all I can tell them is, "I'm sorry, I can't help you." If you can't help them, and they don't want to be referred, then I don't think you do them a favor by keeping them on the hook. I think you can just be perfectly honest with them. "I can't help you." "I'm sorry." Some people you have to tell just this bluntly.

Audience:

This again differs in the situation where you have other physicians there to help them, where you're by yourself and there is no one to easily refer them to. You've got a problem that's a little different than that in a big community where you have someone to help you. This is a real acute problem where we have too many patients and one of these people that they call crocks monopolizes time that you just can't seem to give them. You get frustrated. There comes a limit where either he's got to go or you've got to go. What do you do then?

Dr. Emory:

There are some people who wear you out. I find it depends on who wears out first with some of them. There are some people that I don't take into my consultation room because I can't get rid of them. When I have determined the patient is not organically ill and is not amenable to psychotherapy, I take some protective tactics. Some of them go into the front treatment room so I can get to the back treatment room to my next patient on time. There are some that are just very difficult to handle. But I think sometimes it comes to the point where you just have to sit down and talk to them, straight, as to what the problem is and to state that you are unable to help them under these circumstances, but that if they have a condition in which you can help them then you will be glad to see them. This may open up the psychological problem or may let them know you have not refused to see them. There comes a time when you just have to face the issue and say that you can't manage it. If you're the only physician there, then I don't know where they're going to go. Some people just want an audience and I believe you have to determine whether the doctor's office is the proper place.

Dr. Sorum:

I agree with that, but sometimes they're asking another question. Sometimes what they're asking for is not what they seem to be asking for. I remember two cases. One was a borderline schizophrenic. When I did ask her what was the meaning behind a lot of these things, finally she came out with it. Of course I was dealing with her psychiatrically but she was trying to mediate it all through physical complaints. She couldn't conceive of being ill psychiatrically. She said, "If I get well, you'll really probably never see me again. You know, if I go out and don't have these pains and can go out and get a job, like you say, then there won't be any time for me to come to your office and you

won't be able to take care of me." This is the kind of thing
that sometimes is going on. They're asking for help in a different
way. You sometimes can find out just what language it is they're
talking, and then try to reassure them because their power
struggle develops not about the symptoms, but with the power
struggle with you.

Another one finally told me later, in another moment of
desperation after I'd gone into a rage, as even psychiatrists do,
she said, "You know, when you talk nice to me I get well. When
you get angry, I get sick." What she was telling me there, I
talked to her longer and found out that she was every now and
then testing me by being obnoxious. She'd be obnoxious to see
what I would do. Would I like her if she was that way? If I
liked her, then she would be a little bit less obnoxious.

Dr. Lebensohn:

The case cited by the doctor raises another question and that
is, "What is going on in the life situation which causes hypochondriasis and psychosomatic symptoms to persist?" It reminds
me of the wonderful anecdote attributed to the late Dr. Edward
Weiss, a distinguished Philadelphia internist, who was co-author
with Spurgeon English of that excellent book *Psychosomatic
Medicine*. He told of a woman who had consulted practically
every internist and surgeon in Philadelphia without obtaining
diagnosis or relief. She went from one doctor to another but
continued to get worse and worse. Her skin became sallow, she
lost weight and she became nothing but skin and bones. She
looked like a "hag." It was a ghastly case which stumped the
experts. They thought she might have a hidden carcinoma or
some obscure wasting illness and she was subjected to every test
imaginable. They finally sent her to Dr. Weiss but after a few
visits she stopped coming and he lost track of her. About eight
months after the last visit, Dr. Weiss was walking along Walnut
Street when he saw a very attractive woman walking briskly
toward him. She recognized him immediately and said "You're
Dr. Weiss!" He stopped and said, "Yes. Excuse me, but I do not
know who you are." She replied, "I'm Mrs. so-and-so. Don't
you remember me?" He said, "Well, good heavens! You look

absolutely marvelous. What happened?" She answered, "Don't you know? My husband died!"

Audience:

I'm a flight surgeon. By virtue of a few hours of psychiatric training in our school, we have suddenly become the base psychiatrists. We see a rather exclusive population, but we do have a big problem with these young girls who marry the younger airmen. They live mostly in trailer parks or apartment houses. The suicide attempt rate among these people is just fantastic. I was wondering if there was any way that these could be recognized before they come wheeling into the emergency room after having taken a double handful of something or other. It seems as if they all take pills. The men seem to shoot themselves and the women take pills. Is there any way we could give these people help before they reach this state? Either through educating the other doctors or ourselves, or, in some manner or means, trying to prevent it.

Dr. Ewalt:

You'll have to remember that every suicide, as has been pointed out by various people, has more than one element to it. It's obvious that the person wants to die. He also is angry with somebody and wants to kill somebody. Therefore, it's a display of anger, usually toward a person who has brought about some loss in his life. This is suggestive, therefore, of a great social factor in every suicide, and sometimes it can be picked up. In the situation of the military it has been worse in some of your outlying bases, e.g., some of the Arctic perimeters, etc. I think the approach has to be a matter of education in a group, that is, social support, support of these people in adequate quarters, adequate support for their families and their youngsters. These are things that have to be studied. These people have to have a place they can go, somebody they can confide in. Some of the wives will confide in their friends, and particularly at a time when they've lost their friend, when the husband has gotten irritable or overburdened and troubled himself, and somehow can no longer give the support or has turned his attention away from her.

Sometimes distress arises over transfers that come or transfers that don't come when they're anticipated. Always there's a loss involved somewhere and you have to begin to look for it. You also have to try to work as much as you can in the social setting, although I realize this is almost impossible with military dependents. But it's also very difficult in Roxbury, in Boston, which is to some extent a mixed slum area, to try to give these people outside support, etc. The word should be around that help's available, that there's somebody they can talk to. The chaplains can help, the social workers can help, and if you happen to have psychologists there, they can help. You, yourself, have to do a lot of listening, and you all should be alert to people who begin to withdraw, begin to break off contact with other people, which sometimes happens. They'll no longer want to go out to the bowling league or to the mothers' group or to the sewing group or other kinds of activity. When they begin to withdraw, somebody should look into it and try to find out why. Preachers and school teachers have more authority to go into people's home uninvited and unwanted than anybody else. Doctors can't do this, a lawyer can't, a police officer can't, but a preacher can. Somehow they get away with this kind of thing. A chaplain very often can involve himself in a situation you're worried about, and be looked upon as doing his duty, whereas you'd be nosy if you tried it. I think working out a liaison with them sometimes would help.

Dr. Lebensohn:

Not only would you be nosy but, by your very presence as the base psychiatrist, you would be "tainting" them with the brush of psychiatry. I would like to ask Dr. Key, how many of these young, immature, unhappy women were actually working? Most of them give a history of having worked prior to marriage. Then they marry, leave their job and find that they have nothing to do all day long. Their husbands are involved in their own work and the young wives discover that marriage isn't all it's cracked up to be. They don't have the maturity to make the new adjustment, and so they make a suicidal gesture chiefly to gain attention. (It has been my experience that most women make gestures whereas most men, when they make suicidal attempts, are often successful.)

Again I ask, how many of these patients are working? Very few, I would guess. On a military base it is somehow not considered right to work after marriage. Some of them consider it beneath their dignity to continue to work although work has probably been the only thing that kept them going. A lot of young women decompensate after marriage. They have a lot of starry-eyed, immature and unrealistic ideas of what marriage is all about and, when it doesn't come up to their expectations or when they are frustrated, their frustration tolerance is so low that they take a very easy out. The life history usually reveals that they were very petulant children when they were youngsters and as chronological adults they are really acting out what they did when they were six or seven years old when they couldn't get their way.

Audience:

I'm wondering how deep we should go in our treatment. I've been called out to homes several times when a woman was tearing off her clothes, pulling out her hair, screaming and hollering and evidently needed some sort of treatment. I advised them to send her off to our Florida State Hospital. The next day she'd be perfectly well. But at that particular time she was manic. Evidently the situation corrected itself, but I'm wondering, should we go all out with psychotherapy or just let some things pass over when the immediate situation is over?

Dr. Lebensohn:

This is the sort of question which invariably comes up in a group like this. It's a very important one because of its frequency. The situation seems very clear: what you describe is really a medical and psychiatric emergency. Even if you had a psychiatrist at your elbow, I doubt if he could do any better than you in such a situation. You have phenothiazines and other potent tranquilizers at your command. You now have better chemicals to take care of such acute situations than we have ever had before. Furthermore, you know more about their action than many psychiatrists who see office patients only because you are on the firing line and you see what happens in a real life situation. So the thing to do is to give her a tranquilizer by mouth or by hypo, get some family member, or friend, or nurse to stand by and see what happens. If, after several days of watchful observation the patient doesn't clear up, arrangements can then be made for transfer to a psychiatric hospital.

Dr. Sorum:

Perhaps if you know the history of what she has been doing, what's been leading up to this thing, how many episodes there are, then you can decide whether it's a hysterical episode to gain attention, whether it is manic, or whether it's schizophrenic. There are so many different clues that would be important.

Audience:

I live in a small, rural community, where the people are primarily farmers and ranchers. I can't help but get the feeling where it's indicated they deeply resent any attempt at psychiatric investigation or interviewing. How can you make this more available to the people and make them try to understand what you're trying to do?

Dr. Ewalt:

This is a really tricky question, and a very important one. The same question comes up if you're in an urban area with people from the lower social economic groups, the labor class people, the uneducated people who tend not to conceptualize things in psychological verbal terms. You have to watch out if you're running an institution because, the first thing you know, all your patients are college students—young, attractive, and bright. However, you have to give service to these other people.

We've made various attempts. You have to give them something that they can latch on to. Dr. Lebensohn mentioned this patient from St. Elizabeth's who said it was the hydrotherapy that helped him. When I was down at the University of Texas— the people in Boston are a little more sophisticated and you can't do it, we use tranquilizers now—but down there, to get these people to come in for their prescription and their psychotherapy, I would say, "Now what you need to do is talk to me and tell me about these things, and I'm going to give you a prescription for Vitamin B which you don't need, but at least it won't do you any harm." This was as honest as I knew how to be, and I'd give them the prescription and they would come back the next time for their appointment. "I came in for a new prescription, Doc." They would sit there and talk for whatever I thought they needed—thirty or fifty minutes or whatever—and I would get them to talk about their problems, about themselves, about their cows, and other kinds of things. But they had to have some little excuse for coming, to make it like seeing a doctor. I had to act like a doctor, too, so I gave them these prescriptions for something that they didn't need.

I think, sometimes, that with patients like this you can use a tranquilizer. I have a kind of compulsion about being honest with the patient. When I first tried this I thought it would scare them off. You know, they ignore that. They don't hear it. If you start in and say, "I'm going to give you psychotherapy," this offends almost everybody. If you start in, "I wonder if something is bothering you? What are you worried about? What's making you feel so awful?" they begin to feel that you feel for them and are really interested in them. I don't think they care what you call it.

Dr. Emory:

I'd like to elaborate on that point just a little bit in respect to language, because I think it helps the patient just to put the question to them. You may say, "Well I just don't understand what's going on. Will you tell me? Will you explain it to me?" Let him educate you, and let him do it in his own language. It doesn't have to be psychotherapy or any particular jargon. That's why I think the ear is so important as a therapeutic tool. Let him tell you in his language what he wants to tell you and let him get it off his chest and in terms that he can understand. Then you have a tool with which you can go back to him, and you have the language with which you can go back, too. It doesn't hurt to ask some patients, "What's eating you?"

Audience:

Dr. Lebensohn, not long ago I saw a short spot on television sponsored, I believe, by the State Mental Health Association, about how much help was available now for the alcoholic and I got the distinct impression that the public was being oversold on psychiatric help available, especially in this field. Your statement about not over-selling the patient prompts my question. The question is, how do you feel about advertising mental health programs? Is the public being "oversold" or not being "sold" enough?

Dr. Lebensohn:

You know, a psychiatrist's attitude toward mental health is just the opposite of the clergyman's attitude toward sin. In other words, the clergyman is always *against* sin, and the psychiatrist is always *for* mental health. We are not at all sure what the mental hygiene movement has accomplished. It certainly has not eliminated mental disease. There have been some studies which seem to indicate that the one thing that an active mental health program does do in a small community is to raise the level of anxiety of the population about mental illness. This, it does do, just as a cancer campaign elevates the level of anxiety about cancer. Increased anxiety might be a good thing if it brought people in earlier for treatment. We are not absolutely sure of this in either cancer or mental illness. What has been accomplished is to make going to a psychiatrist somewhat more respectable. It is much more common now than it was twenty-five or thirty years ago. I do not think that the mental health associations or the individual psychiatrists are overselling psychiatry at the moment. In the past, a number of novelists, playwrights and movie makers *did* oversell psychiatry. Fortunately, those days are in the past.

There have been no new breakthroughs in the problem of alcoholism which you mentioned specifically. It's a very serious problem in this country with over five million alcoholics. The attitude of most general hospitals and most general practitioners is, "I don't want to have anything to do with them. They're an unreliable bunch. You can't get them well. What can you do about them?" I think most doctors are getting to the point of referring them to Alcoholics Anonymous which probably has a better record with the alcoholic than any other group.

Dr. Knight:

I want to use the prerogative of the moderator and tell you about a meeting in which I recently took part. There were primarily practitioners in the field of allergy participating. A physician spoke to me and said, "Psychiatry enunciates many principles and you seem to have a great deal of faith in them. For example, the Oedipus Complex—you build a whole system on the concept of the love of mother and son. Why do you pay so much attention to this?" I said, "Actually, psychiatry is built on a very practical wisdom drawn from people and their behavior. For instance, I'll tell you a story that I heard recently that will convince you that there may be some validity in people's concern about the love of son and mother. It seems that this woman was in status asthmaticus and was dying. Her husband had called in all the specialists, and everybody had gotten a crack at treatment, and yet she was still fading fast away. Finally the husband suggested, 'Well, possibly as a final measure why don't we attempt sexual intercourse.' They both thought that was a good idea, so he began this. As he moved along in this type of activity, one bronchiole after another began to relax and she recovered completely. Her color returned and there she was, lying there relaxed and feeling that she would never have asthma again. A few seconds later she looked down and there her husband was sitting at the foot of the bed, crying in an inconsolable fashion. She spoke to him and said, 'Darling, why are you crying? I'm now well. What's wrong?' Through his sobs, he spoke, 'Now I realize I could have saved my mother.'

In closing, I want to mention that I have been impressed by the fact that the speakers have used very little psychiatric jargon and have enunciated very clearly the basic principles involved in patient care and psychiatric treatment. The members of the audience are to be commended for asking relevant and important questions which motivated the splendid discussion. The meeting is adjourned.

THE MEDICAL PRACTITIONER'S MEANS OF COLLECTING PSYCHIATRIC DATA

EDWARD H. KNIGHT, M.D.

THE MOST FREQUENT objection of the general practitioner to psychiatric training is that he simply does not have time to introduce psychotherapeutic measures into his busy practice. To me, this complaint is a valid and self-evident fact. Often practitioners have been urged to set aside a morning or afternoon once a week to see patients with emotional disturbances. I must confess that I used to advocate this system also until I realized that it would, and could, only be used by a few practitioners with a penchant for psychiatry as a subspecialty or a hobby. Moreover, this amount of time could not nearly handle the needs of a large clientele. Also, psychiatric patients and psychiatric principles would become once again sequestered and isolated within their practice. So this would not solve the problem. Instead of bringing psychological awareness into the mainstream of his practice, the GP would only succeed in setting aside a certain portion of his time to be a specialist. Training in psychiatric matters should not have this as its goal. The GP cannot afford to be a part-time psychiatrist any more than he can be a part-time ENT man, radiologist or other specialist.

Psychiatric principles must somehow be brought into the mainstream of everyday general medical practice. To this end the GP must develop his own techniques of observation and intervention, adapted to his particular setting. Psychological principles for the general practitioner will of necessity be somewhat different in their application than those employed by the psychiatrist. The techniques of the psychiatrist are seldom useful or possible for other physicians. For example, the general practitioner can almost never escape an authoritarian role and the consequent dependency that this encourages in his patients. He cannot on one day directly and authoritatively issue instructions regarding physical necessities, and then on the next day sit back in benign psychotherapeutic neutrality requiring that the patient face his own problems and work through decisions in a collaborative, introspective interview. The psychotherapist traditionally avoids advice, instructions, decisions, family contacts, social contact, business relationships and at times office, phone or home visits. The GP would be out of business if he followed suit. These illustrations serve to indicate that psychiatric principles for the GP must be tailored and specially molded to fit the needs of his type of practice as well as the particular type of relationship he must develop with his clientele.

It is therefore worthwhile to attempt some clarification of the medical practitioner's special role as regards his responsibility for the emotional and psychological affairs of his patients. Fundamentally, I think that the GP should make a definite distinction between two broad areas in which psychological principles are applied. The first would be those treatment situations in which an attempt at definitive psychotherapeutic intervention is made; and the second may be termed the incorporation of general psychological principles into everyday office, home and hospital medical procedures and practices. In the first area of definitive psychotherapeutic intervention a medical practitioner may be as good or as poor as his training, inclination and personality attributes will allow. Just as a GP may be particularly facile in one or another specialty, he may also have some knack in psychotherapeutic matters and consequently focus a bit more in this area. Such an effort to help a patient overcome a clearly defined psychiatric illness should only be attempted when the doctor has had sufficient contact, either long term or brief intensive, with the patient so that he may be able to construct a meaningful and useful etiologic formulation. In short, a working hypothesis. If he has known the patient long enough or has been able to spend enough time with the patient he should be able to come to some conclusions regarding first, the basic personality type of the patient, and second the current living stress situation which has produced symptoms. His psychotherapy will be designed to relieve the current stress situation and his responsibility will end there, unless he sees fit to refer the patient on for further treatment designed to affect the basic personality patterns of the individual. He will use drugs, discussion and advice in his effort to relieve symptoms and will encourage insight when possible. If he is unsuccessful in handling the current stress situation he may also find it necessary to make a psychiatric referral.

This brief summary of direct psychotherapeutic intervention is not intended to be exhaustive but to merely clear the way for a discussion of the second major area which is the incorporation of psychological principles into the routine medical procedures of the GP. Here it is my contention that psychiatric principles and concepts must be fitted into and accommodated to the special needs, styles of work and peculiar responsibilities of the medical practitioner. It is generally accepted that the psychological assets and vulnerabilities of the patient are as important as the physiological, hereditary, and other aspects of the total patient picture. As such they should receive no more or less emphasis than the physical features.

Since the GP cannot rely on long interviews, he must accept whatever relationship is available to him in assisting the patient over periodic physical illnesses and also in obtaining his psychiatric data. The psychiatrist in therapy may insist on developing a particular type of clarified, thoroughly discussed relationship. In contrast the medical practitioner may frequently have to accept and work with whatever kind of relationship the patient is able to form. In this sense he is already practicing a highly structured form of psychotherapy. He may at times have to deliberately encourage a dictatorial relationship or perhaps even a hostile one in order to achieve the goals of enforcing a mandatory life or death treatment regime. Relationships for the GP range all the way from friendly and mature to dependent, hostile, suspicious, and at times even completely estranged distant collaboration in the treatment of a part of the patient's body. His advice may be extremely welcome and effective in guiding a patient through emotional crises or it may be totally rejected, the patient feeling that he only wants care for his physical ills and that his emotional life is no one else's business. Therefore, it seems apparent to me that in the ordinary practice of general medicine, the GP must begin by making some effort to determine the nature of his relationship with his patient and not assume that he is expected to offer assistance in psychological matters unless the patient in some way lets him know that this is permissible and desired. Even if it is clear that his patient will only accept physical care, it is still, however, and this I want to emphasize, the doctor's responsibility to be aware of the nature of his relationship to his patient and also to develop as much as an understanding of the patient's personality type as he possibly can. Even though he may never overtly use this information it is still part of his routine continuing observation. To this end I have listed several suggestions for the obtaining of personality and psychological data that I feel may be carried out along with the conventional procedures and techniques of general medical care. This list is of course not complete, not new and each point could be expanded further.

General Relationship

The longer the GP has known a patient the more he should be expected and usually does know about the patient's personality. This increases his responsibility in the event of the emergence of emotional problems. In the course of years and months of contact the practice of recording the patient's responses to instructions, to pain, to illness, to disagreements, to disappointments and to irritations in the medical relationship should be noted, *on the record*. If the relationship has been long it is clear that the doctor is meeting more needs of the patient than simply those that are physical. The doctor should include in his progress notes hints as to why the patient likes him. Is it his skill, his availability, his reputation or his family contacts? A special relationship exists which I have previously labeled as structured and psychotherapeutic. This relationship is an active ingredient of all treatment activity. Therefore, in the interest of objectivity the physician should periodically spell out in writing his delineation of what this relationship is, and is not. Just as careful long range notes regarding physical vulnerabilities will pay off from time to time, the medical practitioner's notations regarding emotional idiosyncrasies will also be of great value when a time of crisis does occur. Most important of all, however, is that in the course of making such personality notations, as a form of discipline, he will inevitably accrue, bit by bit, a far greater understanding of the patient's personality than would otherwise be possible. So often I have noted that physicians' records contain no place for remarks about personality or emotional reactions. In contrast, one GP who does record such observations reported the following anecdote. A patient who through the years always questioned, challenged and criticized treatment measures suddenly and unobstrusively ceased and began to leave the office quietly without comment. At first the GP thought that at last his patient was cooperative. But the contrast was so great that he decided to inquire and found that his seemingly uncomplaining patient was now thoroughly paranoid and obligingly accepting the medicine that he felt was to eliminate him. In this case, definitive psychiatric treatment was begun far sooner than it would have been had the doctor been less astute.

The patient's peculiar and private response to illness offers an excellent opportunity for insights into emotional vulnerabilities and strengths. Does he tend to deny illness or press the panic button with each new symptom? If he is indifferent to physical danger he may be inordinately susceptible to social, occupational and other dangers. In some cases, however, he may be strong in the face of personal, social or financial stresses but crumble and panic under the threat of physical disease. If he comes extremely dependent when frightened by a physical illness, does he lose face and become humiliated after health has been restored? Some patients when well resent the dependency they so desperately sought while ill. Are there any preoccupations about pain and death? Observations made during minor and successfully treated illnesses will prove to be of great value later when the patient is facing serious or more devastating illnesses. On the other hand one may note, if one is interested and makes an effort to observe, that often some patients will experience unusual improvements in personal relationships only when they are ill, and return to their unstable, quarrelsome home life when the illness subsides. All of these observations regarding reaction to illness can be easily obtained during the ordinary course of treating an illness and in fact can only be obtained by the physician who is in attendance at such a time. They offer invaluable insights into the basic personality patterns of each patient. If one takes the trouble to note these reactions he may find his handling of physical illnesses is enhanced, and he will also improve in his ability to guide, advise, predict and anticipate the patient's reactions to future stresses.

Responses to Examinations and Procedures

Responses to examinations and procedures also offer the practitioner a good opportunity to formulate hypotheses and make observations that will allow him to round out his picture of the patient's psychological characteristics. Too often the practitioner long familiar, and even bored, with his innumerable tests and examination devices will forget that each mechanical manipulation is a stimulus to which the patient will respond in a most revealing manner. Patients object to laboratory tests not only for economic reasons but because such procedures often carry magical significance and connote the finding out of something secretly bad or wrong in them. One astute practitioner commented to me that after a battery of tests when he sat down to discuss the results with his patients, he often noted that they seem to feel exposed and opened up like a book. They would have a tendency to want to discuss hidden fears and personal secrets which had not previously been mentioned. This was I think because at such a time the patients felt transparent; that they had been seen through by the tests and, once physical concerns were laid aside, were more than usually predisposed to a discussion of long hidden fears, guilts, secrets and apprehensions. Some patients desire and welcome painful, onerous and troublesome examination procedures as a periodic means of expiation, punishment and in short, masochistic satisfaction. If such a tendency is noted one might be able to predict that under stress an underlying hypochondriasis might emerge. Fear of invasion of body parts by procedures is a well known and often irksome objection that the physician must handle. This, too, can give hints as to not only bodily fears but also emotional conflicts, especially sexual. Opportunities for education or reassurance often arise out of such iatrogenically induced anxieties. The patient who turns himself over willingly and submissively for all sorts of tests and examinations may not be simply cooperative but may be indicating an extreme degree of passivity that will lead to difficult problems of dependency at a later date. It is also well known that patients do not necessarily regard laboratory tests as an evidence of competence on the part of their physician but at times they may see this as a recourse to additional measures because their case is unusual, complicated, difficult or quite serious. Complaining about tests may also be a safe and not to too subtle way of criticizing the doctor.

The Relationship to Relatives

Why not note whether or not the patient comes alone or finds it necessary to come with someone. What particular person does he seem to lean on during times of illness? Or does the patient feel that he can lean on no one when matters of personal health are at stake? If accompanied by a relative does this mean a somewhat less than optimum confidence in the doctor? Some physicians have noted that a patient will bring a certain relative often as a very subtle means of letting the doctor know who is their most troublesome relative. They may bring a relative to do their complaining for them. There are times of course when it may be necessary to work entirely through a capable and interested relative. Do not overlook the possibility that your patient may resent this facile and preferred surrogate. Allowing the patient and his companion to discuss matters in your presence may provide an excellent opportunity to see in living action, some of the very stresses that have been augmenting the illness under treatment.

Relationship to the Physician

One of the most important areas that may be studied is *the patient's method of coming to terms with what the physician has to say to him.* This would include the doctor's resume or explanation of what is wrong and his instructions as to what must be done. The patient who requires a clear comprehensive and thorough exposition of his illness may be demonstrating an excellent capacity to face reality. If this is overdone or there is persistent misunderstanding, it may be that the patient is not accepting and perhaps can never accept the physician's explanation. Only the patient can tell how much truth he can tolerate and he often cannot do this with words. If the patient is satisfied with a few flimsy diagnostic remarks, then one can be sure that he faces other problems in life with a similar superficial effort at denial. If the patient is sophisticated and knowledgeable in medical matters, he may not always be attempting one-up-manship but may simply desire to impress his doctor in the interest of friendship or better treatment.

There are probably few experiences in life more important than the occasion of a physician's diagnostic summation and explanation being offered to a patient. The way in which it is received, assimilated, rejected, mistrusted or avoided offers one of the most excellent opportunities to see the patient's most important emotional mechanisms at work. It is like saying, "I have something extremely important to tell you, *about you.*" What better psychological test is there? The individual's really basic attitudes toward life, self, and others will be revealed on such occasions. Are there any other human reactions more worthy of careful scrutiny and reflection? These things, too, I think should be noted and included in the patient's progress sheet as they will offer a valuable index of the growth or decline of the patient-physician relationship, and the patient's personality itself as time goes on.

All of these observations and perhaps hypotheses regarding the personality traits that are unique and peculiar to each patient should be recorded as data just as we note all other forms of physical or chemical data. Other areas of observation may also be mentioned in passing: the attitude toward hospitalization as an index of fear or need for dependency; reactions to work, to intimate and close emotional ties, toward your other patients seen in the waiting room, your personnel and even your office; the need or longing for a graceful handicap, or in contrast, an intolerance of the least hint that one is anything less than thoroughly potent.

In the aggregate and over a period of time the practice of noting these responses will facilitate the development not only of a thorough knowledge of a particular patient but also of the physician's skill in discerning emotional characteristics. This, in my opinion, will lead the physician to an understanding of his patient far greater than may be obtained by brief psychiatric screening. Such familiarity with the patient's personality will also lead to what I consider the most important dividend that may come from this type of orientation. As I have said, the physician may or may not in his judgment choose, or be able to use, his understanding in the ordinary course of handling his patient's medical problems. In some cases it may greatly facilitate the handling of medical emergencies or ongoing treatments. In other situations he may find his role very limited and even unwanted in areas of emotional conflict. But above and beyond all of this, I think that it places him in a position whereby he, more than any other person, may be on the alert for and able to recognize when an opportunity arises in the patient's life for further significant emotional growth.

It is well known that the occurrence of a serious illness such as a coronary attack, a debilitating, acute illness or a serious permanent handicap may offer an opportunity not just for adaptation and resignation, but also for extensive renovation and reorientation of a person's life.

Patients may be extremely receptive or disposed to attempt significant change in their whole attitude towards themselves, their life, their relationship to others during a time of sickness. The astute physician who has known for years of a chronic emotional maladjustment may find during a serious illness an opportunity to assist the patient in rebuilding a life of more reasonable and appropriate emotional adjustment. I do not say that this is always the case or perhaps even frequently, but I do say that if such a potentiality for significant psychological improvement is present, then it is a physician's responsibility to do more than heal the physical illness but also point his patient in the direction of improved mental functioning This he will be able to do if he has throughout the years taken the trouble to note carefully the patient's personality traits and emotional vulnerabilities. Just as he would seize the initiative when the opportunity arose to assist his patient in matters of physical hygiene he should also be alert to the opportunities for improvement in mental hygiene.

In conclusion I cannot resist the temptation to respond to another of the medical practitioners' frequent and justifiable questions —or perhaps complaints—that is, "What do I do?" It must be clear that I have not mentioned anything that should be done except to observe, to speculate, to formulate hypotheses and to record them. This in brief is the very thing that the psychiatrist does in his treatment. This is psychotherapy. As the process of attentive observation, reflective formulation and broadened awareness proceeds, so too does understanding of the patient proceed. Understanding in the doctor is the *sine qua non* of understanding in the patient himself about himself. There are no magical interpretations, no substitutes, for enlightened acceptance and knowledge of what makes a person feel and think the way he must. Your patient can only know and forgive himself when you can. This is treatment, and this is the rationale behind my exhortation to observe, study and note your patient's behavior when and where it occurs. Treatment is not telling a patient how he should think or feel, but helping him understand how he does feel and think. You can only do this when you have utilized the rich potentialities of the medical relationship, to the fullest, in understanding him.

A NEW LOOK AT ALCOHOLISM

PHILIP SOLOMON, M.D.

F OR CENTURIES, ALCOHOLISM has been looked upon as a form of evil-doing, comparable to and often associated with drug addiction, gambling, and various forms of criminality. In recent years, it has become fashionable to consider alcoholism as "illness" rather than "badness." While much good has resulted from this change as far as the fate of many individuals afflicted with alcoholism is concerned, little progress has been made toward the better scientific understanding of the basic conditions involved. Our ignorance regarding alcoholism is essentially as abysmal today as it was in the days of Hippocrates.

The truth may well be that there is no one "cause" of alcoholism but that the condition will have to be looked upon as a form of behavior which may be brought about through the action of any one of several factors: physiological, psychological, or sociological. Badness and illness may be involved individually, or together, or not at all. There may be no two cases exactly alike.

At Boston City Hospital, problems of alcoholism are rampant. About half our patients throughout the hospital, in-patients and out-patients, present themselves with alcoholism either as a primary or secondary cause of their difficulties. Acute and chronic alcoholic intoxication, alcoholic gastritis, pancreatitis, cirrhosis of the liver, multiple peripheral neuritis, encephalopathies, various other associated avitaminoses, Wernicke's disease, Korsakoff's psychosis, degeneration of the cerebellum, delirium tremens, rum fits, hallucinosis, dementias—all of these and many combinations abound in our hospital. When the Psychiatry Service was organized (scarcely more than a decade ago), it was clear from the outset that our chief field for attention and inquiry should be alcoholism.

Our early studies were largely clinical and exploratory. We tabulated the attitude of our physicians toward the alcoholic patient (1) and noted the correlation of punitivism with authoritarianism. We described a collection of unusual "super-alcoholics," for whom ordinary ethyl alcohol was too mild and who became addicted to one or another of the higher, more toxic, alcohols (2). We investigated magnesium levels in delirium tremens (3), tested a new therapeutic preparation in this disorder (4), and studied the differentiation of delirium tremens from impending hepatic coma (5). We soon decided that definitive progress in the understanding of alcoholism would probably not be made until crucial experimental work could be carried out on alcoholic patients themselves.

Our first experimental objective, carried out by my associate, Dr. Jack Mendelson and assistants, was to throw light on the *physiological components* of alcoholism by investigating tissue tolerance, physical dependency, and withdrawal phenomena as indicators of the *addiction factor* (6). Volunteer subjects who were chronic alcoholics and who had previously experienced delirium tremens were given increasing amounts of alcohol every four hours around the clock until they were receiving forty ounces of 86 proof whiskey every twenty-four hours. After a twenty-four-day period of drinking they were abruptly stopped. Eight out of ten developed acute withdrawal symptoms (tremor, orientation and memory deficits, and hallucinations) within twenty-four hours of the last dose of alcohol.

A number of physiological parameters were studied in this experiment and the following additional findings are of interest: the subjects suffered gastritis during the experiment (nine of ten), but there was no liver damage or loss of weight. Protein appeared in the urine in the last stages of the experiment (nine of ten), but disappeared promptly when drinking ceased. Ketonuria (ten of ten) and glucosuria (four of ten) also disappeared dramatically at the end of the experiment. Serum uric acid, glycerides, phospholipids, free fatty acids, and cholesterol all rose during the alcohol phase and returned to control levels after withdrawal. Serum magnesium was unchanged until after withdrawal, and it then declined significantly. Serum glucose was unchanged throughout.

Psychologically, there was an increase rather than a decrease in feelings of anxiety in the subjects as drinking progressed. There was little aberrant behavior: one subject became depressed and one paranoid, both only for a few days. Social interaction among the group was high and mutual concern was exhibited. At the maximum dosage, further increase of anxiety was accompanied by the development of aggressiveness, and craving for alcohol was manifested, but was associated with ambivalence. Motor performance, reaction time, and attention were not impaired at 30 oz. of whiskey a day, but were at 40. Brain waves showed slowing of alpha frequencies but a rapid return to normal on withdrawal.

With regard to ethical considerations in this experiment, it should be noted that participation was entirely voluntary, every effort was made to minimize hazards, and all subjects were offered long-term therapy following the end of the study. Actually, the relationships that were developed during the study turned out to be of great value in constructing a beneficial therapeutic alliance with these subjects, so that they did well later.

The chief conclusion to be drawn from the above experiment is that, under the conditions given, physical dependence of *addiction to alcohol* does take place. Much work remains to be done to elucidate, with respect to alcoholic addiction, its prevalence, conditions for production, degrees of severity, manner of quantification, dangers, and proper management. We are proceeding with some of the problems involved by employing radioactive alcohol (tagged with carbon-14), in order to study metabolic aspects of alcohol utilization and degradation.

Our next concern at Boston City Hospital has been to investigate the *psychological components* in alcoholism, as indicators of the *habituation factor,* or *craving.* Here, Dr. Mendelson and Dr. Nancy Mello have been working out an ingenious operant conditioning technique which provides an objective measure of an individual's desire for alcohol in terms of the amount of work he is willing to do to get it. An elaborate machine device is programmed to reward the subject, after he has accomplished the necessary and correct amount of work on its various colored buttons, with either a shot of whiskey or a plastic token which later can be exchanged for whiskey. A measure of the subject's ability to delay receiving the reward (and thus the urgency of his craving) is furnished by the circumstance that removing the cup from the machine in order to drink its contents breaks a circuit and causes a delay of several minutes before the subject can begin working again for more whiskey. Monitoring the subject's drinking behavior and studying it in conjunction with objective records of his ward behavior provide a method of investigating the all-important factor of psychological motivation in alcoholism. When baselines are established, the effects of drugs, psychotherapy and other techniques of management will then be susceptible to scientific scrutiny and reproducible manipulation. This work is now in progress.

After objective and quantitative measures are available for the evaluation of both the addictive and craving factors in the alcoholic population, the work on the *sociological component* will be a much simpler job. All three components—physiological, psychological, and sociological—must yield to scientific analysis before alcohol can return to its rightful place of being a boon and not a bane to mankind.

TREATMENT

A clinician usually cannot wait for a full scientific understanding of his patient's trouble before undertaking to treat it. A suffering human being must be helped by whatever means are at hand, be they entirely pragmatic or based on trial and error. In the case of chronic alcoholism, much experience, not all happy, is at our disposal.

If you are trying to rescue someone who is drowning, the first thing you want to do is to get him out of the water. Even before you do any artificial respiration or anything else you just have to get him out of that water. This is one thing that is equally true of rescuing an alcoholic patient. It is imperative to get him out of his atmosphere of drinking. The problem is not so much one for the physician or psychiatrist, but one for sociologists, friends, clergymen, and ancillary workers without whom we just cannot appropriately deal with the problem of alcoholism. The familiar team of psychiatrist, psychologist, and social worker is valuable in the treatment of alcoholic patients. In private practice one does not have to have these assistants. One can do a good deal by oneself, but the approach has to be the same. You must take cognizance of the fact that your patient, if he goes back to his familiar environment where he is associated with his cronies who do all the drinking, will continue to drink in spite of all your best efforts in your office. The primary emphasis has to be laid on the matter of doing something about the patient's social environment. Usually this must be done through the family, if there is a family. Many of these people, by the time you see them, have long since alienated themselves from their family. If not by them, then by some organization such as Alcoholics Anonymous. AA is extremely helpful with many of our patients and we urge you to keep it in mind and to try it in cases where you do not have direct help from other social agencies. With regard to the family, one of the most important things to emphasize is they must be tolerant and patient and cooperative, even when the patient has relapses. It is perfectly all right for them to condemn the drinking, but not the drinker. This must be true of the physician, as well. Even your condemnation of his drinking has to be carefully stated. You must refrain from being outspokenly censorious. The subject must feel that you are for him, that you are on his side.

A good way to establish this relationship of your being on his side is to start with something in the realm of the physiology of the individual—his physical make-up. In each instance, a very careful, unusually detailed physical examination should be done. This patient must have the feeling that you are sincerely interested in him and in his body. Do all the neurological tests. Do anything that you can to determine if there is physical and neurological damage, but more importantly to convince him of the thoroughness with which you are attempting to help him. You almost invariably will find something physical that you can do something about. He may have bad teeth or need new glasses or have constipation or some varicose veins or hemorrhoids.

It is important to find something that you can help physically. Then you are off to a great start, and he is on your side and he feels that you are really out to help him.

The same attitude should be taken towards intellectual approaches. Something should be done towards enlisting his intellect, his mind. Something that makes him feel that you are determined to make him a better man. Somehow you must find a way to convince him that he has been underestimating himself, which he usually has been, and that you respect him and that he should respect himself. This is the principle of it. How you do it will be an individual matter concerned with your own special techniques and with the kind of a man you are dealing with. You must show him that he can respect himself better than he is, that he can do more in life than he has been doing, and that he has got a future that is a lot better than he thought it was.

You must not neglect the spiritual, either. The patient can want to stop drinking in one sense, but not in another. One alcoholic patient came staggering into his doctor's office, obviously very drunk and said, "Doctor, I've succeeded in triumphing over my will power!" The will power is the problem. Sure, they all want to stop drinking, at least so they tell you. But later they want more to drink and there are different levels in the conscience, or superego, that constitute the problem. You know, they say the superego is that part of the mental apparatus that is soluble in alcohol. Indeed it often seems just like that. Once they start drinking their desire not to drink vanishes. But, as I say, these are the factors that we know so little about and we are trying to learn more about. Nevertheless, you should try to work with his spiritual make-up (I don't know if you would insist on saying that this is different from his psychological or mental make-up). If a man has something that is important to him—religious beliefs, principles, philosophical view of life—enlist these in support of your treatment. This can sometimes be done through his religious advisor, priest, minister, rabbi. It can be done through friends who may still be interested in him or relatives. It can be done through the man, himself.

I should say one word about your own attitude. You must learn to be terribly, terribly patient and tolerant and not overambitious with what your treatment is going to do. Alcoholics notoriously have relapses. They constantly make great promises, and mean them when they make them, and then find themselves undermined later and unable to keep their promises. You must not condemn a relapse. You cannot do that without losing the feeling that the patient is still joined with you in the treatment. You must stay with him, no matter what happens, as patiently as you can. This will sometimes be a great strain on you. You must avoid the feeling of megalomania that too many of us have, expecting that just because we want the patient to do something he will. You must wear your halo gracefully. But if a doctor persists with an alcoholic and stays with him, then I feel that the general practitioner, or any non-psychiatrist physician, can do just as well as any of our alcoholic clinics do or any of our psychiatrists. How do we do? The standard results are one-third cured, one-third somewhat better, one-third unchanged. You can do that just as well as we can and I strongly urge you to try.

Let me add a few more comments drawn from experience at Boston City Hospital. Let us divide chronic alcoholism into three main types, using the criteria already referred to in discussing the rationale for our research efforts, but embodying them in diagnostic categories which are familiar clinically. *Psychosocial* alcoholism will refer to those individuals whose drinking is primarily a pattern of behavior adopted as a means of conforming to the accepted social group. The aim is peer approval. *Psychoneurotic* alcoholism will include the large number of human beings for whom drinking fulfills a persistent neurotic need. The aim is relief from anxiety or the establishment in some other psychodynamic way of greater emotional homeostasis. *Psychotic* alcoholism will designate patients whose alcoholic bouts represent psychotic equivalents, that is to say, substitutes or masks for episodes of psychosis, for example, depression, hypomania, catatonic excitement, or schizophrenic dissociation. The aim is desperate escape from what seems like imminent dissolution, annihilation, or dispair.

The three types are not mutually exclusive or statistically fixed. One spree drinker whose violent episodes of alcoholism usually represent eruptions of repressed sadistic rage and fury, also drinks occasionally to be "one of the boys." Another alcoholic began to drink because all the members of his gang did, but after several years, he is married, living in another city, and is found now to be drinking as a reaction to unconscious feelings of inferiority. A woman who used to drink before going out on social engagements in order to overcome her feelings of shyness now drinks heavily to deny profound depression.

Addiction may occur in any type if there is prolonged indulgence. It is rare in the relatively pure psychosocial alcoholics even after several years of drinking. A fundamental change of scene and a reasonably healthy personality makeup can bring about abstinence without a sign of withdrawal symptoms. Addiction is more common in prolonged psychoneurotic alcoholism, perhaps because the condition is more common and persists longer. In psychotic alcoholics* addiction does not occur if the sprees are far apart and of short duration, but may if they are long and drawn out. What has been said about addiction applies equally to *habituation*, though in the latter the correlation is more clearly one with duration of drinking whereas in the former a hypothetical constitutional or predisposing factor sometimes seems to be operating.

In many cases, regardless of type, years and years of drinking seem to bring about a state of physical, psychological, and moral degradation which results in an end-product which is hard to distinguish one from another. This is the "skid-row" type of chronic alcoholic, usually severely habituated and addicted, devoid of much individualization in personality, lacking in will power or strength of character, homeless, friendless, penniless and destitute, living only for alcoholic oblivion. Such alcoholics are already almost as much alike as cadavers.

In *psychosocial* alcoholism, the main emphasis in treatment should be to manipulate the environment in some favorable way.

---

* The expression "psychotic alcoholic" or "psychotic drinker" here designates an individual who suffers from "psychotic alcoholism." He is not simply an alcoholic who happens also to be psychotic at the time. He is still a "psychotic alcoholic" between bouts, even when not actually psychotic or alcoholic at the time. This is true in the same way that an "alcoholic" is considered to be such even when he may have been abstinent for years.

The psychiatric social worker, AA, vocational counselor, or other agency workers should be enlisted heavily. A new home or job may be the vital change that will make all the difference.

In *psychoneurotic* alcoholism, your own contact and the psychotherapy you do with the patient will be crucial. This is not the place to discuss the details of psychotherapy for busy physicians, but those of you who are interested are urged to look into a recent book by Tedesco (7).

In *psychotic* alcoholism, organic and physical treatments must be resorted to. In the schizoid and dissociated states, where alcoholic sprees represent a kind of schizophrenic break-through (or defense against it, or a bit of *each*), hospitalization, psychiatric consultation, and usually large doses of one of the phenothiazines (Thorazine®, Mellaril®, Stelazine®) are indicated. In the depressive equivalents, where a man drinks desperately because he senses a dangerous depression is threatening to overcome him, again hospitalization and psychiatric consultation must be arranged. If a suicide attempt is considered imminent, electroshock treatments should then be given. Otherwise one of the more rapidly acting and effective antidepressant drugs (Elavil®, Tofranil) should be administered.

In conclusion, let me say that the treatment of alcoholism, in essence, is the same as that for any other disease. Learn what you can of its causes—here they will be sociological, physiological, and psychological—and do what you can to eliminate them or modify them specifically. In addition, use nonspecific treatment to boost the defenses of nature in the patient—through helping him socially, physically, emotionally, and spiritually.

REFERENCES

1. Mendelson, J. H., Wexler, D., Kubzansky, P. E., Harrison, R., Leiderman, G., and Solomon, P.: Physicians' attitudes toward alcoholic patients. *Arch. Gen. Psychiat., 11*:392-399, 1964.
2. Mendelson, J. H., Wexler, D., Leiderman, P. H., and Solomon, P.: A study of addiction to nonethyl alcohols and other poisonous compounds. *Quart. J. Stud. Alcohol, 18*:561-580, 1957.
3. Mendelson, J. H., Wexler, D., Kubzansky, P., Leiderman, P. H., and Solmon, P.: Serum magnesium in delirium tremens and alcoholic hallucinosis. *J. Nerv. Ment. Dis., 128*:352-457, 1959.

4. Wexler, D., Leiderman, P. H., Mendelson, J. H., Kubzansky, P., and Solomon, P.: The effect of cetadiol on delirium tremens, alcoholic hallucinosis, and alcohol withdrawal. *Amer. J. Psychiat.*, *114*:935-936, 1958.

5. Davidson, E. A., and Solomon, P.: The differentiation of delirium tremens from impending hepatic coma. *J. Ment. Scie.*, *104*:326-333, 1958.

6. Mendelson, J. H., *et al.*: Experimentally induced chronic intoxication and withdrawal in alcoholics. *Quart. J. Stud. on Alcohol*, Supplement No. 2, 1964.

7. Castelnuovo-Tedesco, Pietro: *The Twenty-minute Hour*. Boston, Little, Brown, 1965.

DEPRESSIVE REACTIONS TREATABLE BY MEDICAL PRACTITIONERS

GENE L. USDIN, M.D.

SOME CLINICIANS MAINTAIN that the most common symptom seen in the practice of medicine is anxiety. While anxiety may be the most frequent complaint, the most frequent causative factor in complaints is depression. We all recognize the typical symptoms of anxiety—palpitation, tachycardia, hyperhidrosis, feeling of apprehension or alarm, and numerous others. While we recognize the typical mood of a depressive, we do not take into account the numerous routes that a depression may take—the masked, denied or unrecognized depression. What may also be a factor is that patients speak more readily of their anxiety and tension and of alarm and fear than they do of their being sad or depressed. Perhaps the physician does not like to hear that his patient is depressed. It may either stir up feelings within himself, or it may be "too psychiatric." My contention is that for a variety of reasons the physician frequently not only does not inquire regarding depressed feelings, but too often does not consider depression as a possibility. Perhaps the nonpsychiatric physican feels inadequate to deal with a depression. Maybe there is a deficit in the physician's knowledge of the handling and treatment of depressions.

Any physician should be able to recognize psychotic depressions. Too many physicians have problems in appreciating or recognizing nonpsychotic depressions.

This paper concerns the recognition and treatment of depression not so much by specialized psychiatric techniques as by techniques appropriate for medical practitioners.

Depression and anxiety are frequently associated. Depressed feelings are something that all of us have encountered many times within ourselves. All of us have, at times, had enough depression that one could say we had an element of a clinical depression. It is the emotional symptom that our close friends will confide to us most frequently at cocktail parties or other social functions. Actually, only about 25 percent of depressed patients reach the psychiatrist. The vast majority are seen, and should be seen and handled, by the medical practitioner.

Treatment of any medical condition first stems from the recognition of the condition with which one is dealing. Awareness of the current therapy and prognosis is basic. Physicians would do well to develop more acumen in the diagnosis of minor depressions. As has been mentioned, many depressions are masked. It is surprising how often the physician fails to attempt to elicit symptoms that would reveal a depression. Some of the more valuable diagnostic clues that can be put together to form a symptom complex are the vegetative signs and symptoms. All of these should be inquired about in the routine examination.

What are these vegetative signs and symptoms? A list would include: chronic fatigue, anorexia, weight loss, insomnia, decreased or absent sexual desire, constipation; and in more severe depressions, amenorrhea or oligomenorrhea. When one encounters a few of these vegetative symptoms, he should become aware of the depth of the depression—aware that any depressive can commit suicide—and consider the patient medically or psychiatrically ill. In my experience, the earliest of these symptoms are insomnia, anorexia and decreased sexual desire. Constipation seems to be present only in the more severe depressions, and not always even then. Before one lends credence to the symptom of constipation, however, he has to confirm that the constipation has not been present over a long period of time. I recall the late Dr. John Herr Musser saying that one of the sure things that you could know about a woman who has had children was that she would be constipated.

In the literature, amenorrhea and oligomenorrhea are mentioned much more than I seem to find it in my practice. Here again, when present because of a depression, it occurs in those with severe psychopathology. Amenorrhea can provide a complication in that the patient may think she is pregnant and have the emotional reaction secondary to her feelings about pregnancy. This can be a diagnostic problem and sometimes you will do well to confirm by laboratory tests whether or not the patient is pregnant, whether it is a symptom of a depressive reaction, or whether some other condition is causing the amenorrhea.

Sometimes the physician has been told by the family that the patient is severely depressed, cries profusely and has become withdrawn. The patient may deny this. He may cover up his depressed mood and feelings. Still others may be having a smiling depression. In the absence of depressive content, questioning them about vegetative symptomatology can become a valuable diagnostic tool. Sometimes the patient may be a lifelong severe neurotic who has always embroidered his complaints. Here, absence of vegetative symptomatology may serve somewhat as a criteria. On the other hand, the patient may be a chronic depressive and exacerbation of the vegetative symptomatology may alert us to the possibility that he is getting worse.

Dr. Ewalt has discussed physical complaints that may be due to a depression. Patients mask depressions not only from the physician, but also from themselves. They may have no awareness that beneath their discomfort and complaints is a depressive reaction. They come in with aches and pains in various parts of their body that are most genuine insofar as they are concerned. We often find various anxiety symptoms with depression—palpitation, tachycardia, nausea, globus hystericus. These symptoms are often involved in depressions and sometimes they are not obvious anxiety symptoms.

A most important psychic manifestation that should be considered is suicidal ideation. This must always be thought of in any depression, but it is too frequently not considered. Some have the misconception that to question the patient about suicide might put the idea in the patient's mind. This is an unfortunate misconception. It will not strengthen the idea of suicide. It may aid the patient in talking about it and give him a better appreciation that the physician can understand what he is experiencing. This somewhat relieves many patients and also the serious or determined ones may become more evident or reveal themselves.

The physician's role in dealing with a possible suicide may be emphasized by reminding ourselves that many patients who successfully commit suicide while in a depressed condition had the potential and probability of living happy, effective, productive lives. Most who unsuccessfully attempt suicide are regretful thereafter for having tried. Exceptions may be the attention seekers in whom the attempt is mainly an effort to acquire secondary gains.

Many misconceptions are present about the potentiality of suicide. These include the fallacy that religious beliefs are an effective check. Priests, ministers and rabbis have committed suicide. In considering the three major faiths in this country, the one that most clearly establishes suicide as a mortal sin is the Catholic faith. However, it is interesting to note that the lowest rate of suicide is not among Catholics, but among Jews. Other misconceptions concern the idea that those who talk about suicide will never do it, that children will not commit suicide, and that mental defectives will not commit suicide.

Statistics regarding suicide are intriguing. Whereas three times as many females as males attempt suicide, there are three times as many successful suicides by males as females. There is no accepted definite explanation. The mode of execution may be an explanation in that males are more prone to attempt suicide by violent means, for example gunshots or jumping from high buildings, whereas females are more prone to utilize gas and ingestion of sedatives. The male's personality is more action oriented than the females. Also females more frequently have a hysterical personality and a suicide attempt is another means of attempting to get more attention. On any large hospital service, a large number of unsuccessful suicide attempts are by hysterics. Another important point which we need bear constantly in mind is that serious chronic disease or severe pain is depressing and may result in suicide. In large general hospitals there are more suicides on the nonpsychiatric services than on the psychiatric services.

Another interesting finding is that while we are prone to think of paranoid personalities as homicidal, they also have an increased suicidal potential. A physician seeing a suspicious, hostile, aggressive patient talking about self-harm should heed this patient more carefully in appreciating that the potential of self-harm is greater. The paranoid patient may feel trapped, beaten or cornered by his delusions, and if he cannot attack may kill himself—or he may commit suicide to escape spiritual or mystical persecution.

There are two million suicide attempts annually in this country, so it is something with which physicians have to deal. Many of us are not perceptive of warnings sent out by depressed persons—warnings that the patient might commit or attempt to commit suicide.

Evaluation of the depth of a depression is an area that reminds one that medicine remains an art rather than a science, for the ability to evaluate the depth still depends upon the clinical experience and judgment of the physician. There are adjuncts one uses in evaluation such as slow movements, restlessness, facial expression and body posture. One should also be concerned if the patient has become more apathetic, lost interest or has become more introverted. Physicians should take cognizance of the mood and thought content of the patients. Are they preoccupied with anything? One of the cardinal danger signs is when the patient starts expressing feelings of worthlessness, inadequacy, uselessness or "badness." No amount of reassurance from physicians and friends can overcome these feelings in severely depressed persons. It may in fact intensify guilt. Quite frequently the patient projects all of his depressed feelings on having made a poor financial deal—of having been "taken." What he actually is doing is focusing on some happening or transaction as a cause for his low self-esteem and feelings of inadequacy. Quite often one sees a patient who has purchased a home and become convinced that he overpaid for that home. His reaction may be quite disproportionate to his financial disaster. The physician needs to discuss not so much the business transaction but instead the patient's present general concept of himself.

Guilty feelings deserve special emphasis. Guilt is often

related to hostile feelings that the patient has toward others and cannot express or tolerate. Many times these hostile feelings are unconscious or even introjected. This is why it is so important to differentiate grief as a normal reaction from depression as a pathological one. If a person loses a loved one or a loved object, it is appropriate to be upset and to cry. It is appropriate not to want to mingle and not to be gregarious. The individual has lost a love object, and it takes a certain working through of a grief reaction for individuals to reestablish their equilibrium. If you find a person who has lost someone close to him and he seems to have no reaction, you might have more concern than if he is undergoing some type of grief reaction. What often happens is that on a level that is not conscious to patients, there are guilt feelings which they must deny, and later, whether it is two or three months and seemingly unrelated to the loss of the supposed love object, we find the depressive reaction entering in. If the grief reaction lasts too long or is too intense, then we call it a pathological depressive reaction.

Depression should be looked on as a self-punitive mechanism. In a way, it is as if the individual himself is slowly dying, especially if we recall just what the vegetative symptomatology or physiologic decline is in this condition—a slowing of life processes. The grief work is the gradual acceptance of the fact that the love object is lost and that the lost love object must be replaced by something else. This substitute may be another person, several persons, a cause—something to get involved in—a goal. Again, it is appropriate for a person to feel sad, to lose some interest, but there are limits to which a person should have this loss of interest.

It is unnecessary to hospitalize a patient with a grief reaction. He may be depressed for a few days, but there are none of the apparent danger signs. It is amazing what you can accomplish if you can go in with these persons—and this is where I think the medical practitioner can do effective therapy—and provide them with a sympathetic, permissive but objective attitude. The person in a depressive reaction—here we are thinking of guilt—will not talk much about his relative, will not say how much he misses him, how he loved him and how wonderful he was. I think it is quite appropriate for a physician at this time to say, "Well, we all sometimes have some harsh feelings toward our father or mother or wife, and sometimes we feel guilty about this." This maneuver utilizes the concept of universalization. The patient very often will say, "No, I do not have any harsh feelings. I never did feel hostile or guilty about my father or mother. No, there was nothing I should have done in the last few weeks or few months that I now regret." I strongly believe it behooves a physician who, when he feels that this grief reaction is inappropriate, and is building up to something more, to universalize these feelings. No one loves anyone else 100 per cent. We all have ambivalence towards our love objects. Every one of us at some time resents our sons, daughters and wives, and they reciprocate this. This is part of all normal relations. If, as a physician, we can show acceptance, we can accomplish a great deal. Universalization tends to dilute, spread and rationalize the guilt, but it does permit awareness of resentment.

What else should the physician keep in mind regarding the diagnosis of a depression? Certainly here, as in other fields of medicine, the patient's previous history is of cardinal importance. Has the patient ever had a depression or attempted suicide before? Once having attempted suicide, the patient has a much greater probability of attempting suicide again than someone who has never attempted it.

What is the basic personality or neurotic diathesis of the individual? Especially, how is his self-esteem? Is he hypersensitive, too introspective or too introverted?

One finding that I think is overemphasized is that depressions are worse in the morning. Depressives *usually* feel worse in the morning, but we may be overemphasizing this. A large number of depressives get more depressed late in the afternoon following or anticipating situational provocations. Some persons don't get depressed while they have enough to keep them occupied. Others get depressed when they have time to think or are left alone. The most frequent explanation for depression being worse in the early morning is that life basically is so unpleasant for these persons that they dread the prospect of facing the entire day. On the other hand, some depressives frequently sleep fitfully, if at all, and this can be a factor.

Depressives may also be depressing. I recall an incident when I was a psychiatric ward officer at the San Diego Naval Hospital in 1947. A boot class seaman was being surveyed out of the service to a Veterans Administration facility. He was one of the saddest persons I have seen. I called the intern and said, "Dr. Brown, this man is leaving in two days. You have nothing to do this afternoon. Just go over and cheer him up." Dr. Brown was a fine physician, sensitive, competent and jolly. In less than ten minutes Dr. Brown returned. He was actually sobbing. He said, "I can't stand it any longer." Perhaps that was too much empathy or overidentification.

What cannot be emphasized enough is that the family physician is in a better position to aid the patient than would be a new figure, the psychiatrist. If you can give first aid, it can be good aid. If the non-psychiatric physician is at all uncertain about the suicide potential or severe mental illness, he can arrange for psychiatic consultation. Often when a psychiatrist sees a patient in a mild depression, he can recognize that the referring physician is able to handle the problem and probably will be better accepted by the patient. After all, you are introducing a new element, a stranger. If you have had a good relationship with your patient, are aware of your limitations and are willing to give the necessary time, you may be able to do a lot more than the psychiatrist. A psychiatrist has to embark on an entirely new course of treatment and begin a new and unfamiliar relationship. After all, the *sine qua non* of any therapeutic relationship is the interpersonal relationship between the patient and the doctor. This relationship is not established in the first or second visit. When we apparently get that relationship in the first or second visit, we should be alerted to the fact that it isn't a genuine transference of feelings from the patient to us—that there is something unhealthy about it. If the patient comes in at the end of the second visit and says, "Well Doctor, I trust you completely. You are the greatest. I know you can help me," beware of a magical, unrealistic, overvalued relationship. If you have been a good family physician, a good medical practitioner, the patient doesn't have to say that because both of you will know it.

There are so many misconceptions that seem to arouse guilt in our culture, in our society, in our patients. Our culture tends to make one guilty about hostile feelings. One shouldn't have status wishes. One shouldn't have envy. Sometimes it is very good therapy for the physician to acknowledge to the patient that we all have certain status needs, we all get envious, and certain things make all of us feel guilty. Again, universalization is frequently a wonderful technique. We can say, "Well, we all have certain problems. However, you are the patient. Let's talk about yours today." The important point for the physician, again, is to help the patient realize that most of his feelings are not unique or different from others. It is important for the patient to realize that in spite of superficial facades, there is present in all of us a need to be loved, a need to lean on someone, and a need to be taken care of in a childlike, protected fashion. Sometimes our mates do not fulfill these needs when we require them.

Many individuals harbor within themselves awareness of some neurotic traits, overemphasizing the significance of these traits, and feeling that they are in danger of a nervous breakdown. It becomes very important for the depressive to learn that all individuals have neurotic traits and that we differ only in the degree to which we manifest or feel these traits. Patients relate events, happenings, or thoughts to which they attach much anxiety or guilt, in spite of the fact that these traits, or happenings, may be a generally normal development of the personality. Every once in a while a patient says, "Well Doctor, I want to tell you something. It has been difficult for me to say this." Then as he starts discussing the problem, he seems to stop halfway. One waits for the climax wherein he deviates so much from normal. Sometimes the physician says, "Well, have you finished? Have you reached your guilty point?" Again, universalization is important in accepting some of our problems and inadequacies.

Utilization of specific drugs is to be covered in tomorrow morning's session. There is considerable question about the efficacy of antidepressant drugs. We know that there is a strong correlation between the physician's confidence in the drugs and the efficacy. Antidepressant drugs certainly have value and there is every reason to believe that more effective ones will continue to be discovered. It may be that antidepressant drugs are being prescribed too casually and indiscriminately. When an antidepressant drug is prescribed, individual dosages must be established, good contact with a patient should be maintained, and the physician should be aware of and alert to side effects. We may have overplayed avoiding barbiturates because of their depressant effect as insomnia is frequently a prominent symptom that results in many other symptoms. It becomes important to aid the patient with this problem. The shorter-acting barbiturates can be quite helpful for sleep, and if properly prescribed usually will not be depressing.

To conclude—the nonpsychiatric physician must remain aware of the importance of his role in the treatment of depressives. Some have innate ability regarding psychotherapy. Unfortunately, some adopt too much omniscience or omnipotence when they practice psychotherapy. When referral to a psychiatrist is indicated, the manner of referral is of major importance to the ultimate success of therapy.

PANEL DISCUSSION

MODERATOR: MOTTRAM TORRE

PANELISTS: KNIGHT, SOLOMON, AND USDIN

Dr. Torre:

We HAVE LISTENED with great interest to the presentations this morning. We have heard that almost one half of the patients seen by the general practitioner suffer from alcoholism or have conditions that are complicated by the excessive use of alcohol. We have also heard that half of the patients seen by psychiatrists suffer from a primary depression or a psychiatric illness exhibiting depression as one of its symptoms. We must, therefore, conclude that either most of the patients are suffering from either depression or alcoholism, or that the combination of depression and alcoholism occurs quite frequently. I hope that the panelists will discuss this.

Alcohol is a drug that has been readily available to most people in most communities for many years. Many people do use it as a drug. Dr. Solomon indicated that his research demonstrated that it is not a very good tranquilizer for relieving the anxiety in his patients. Yet, it is very extensively used as a tranquilizer. With the recent development of more effective tranquilizers, we now can frequently successfully substitute them for alcohol in patients who are using alcohol as a tranquilizer, and getting into difficulties because of the other effects of alcohol.

Dr. Solomon:

The statement I made had to do not with patients, but with chronic alcoholics who were experimentally given alcohol. My statement was that in these individuals, alcohol did not decrease their anxiety, but actually increased it as the experiment went on. That statement doesn't at all apply necessarily to non-alcoholics and their use of alcohol. It may be that any of us here might find that under conditions of stress and strain, alcohol would help us and would diminish our anxiety, and I would not by any means be surprised if this were the case.

May I just proceed a little. One of you in the audience asked me during the coffee break about the kind of alcoholic who goes on compulsive binges. There certainly are patients who go on terrific binges and seem to drink compulsively. My comment was that this is the kind of patient who may very well be using alcoholism as a mask for depression. We do find quite a number of individuals who are essentially manic-depressive in their make-up, who instead of getting depressed, go into a severe alcoholic binge and the one takes the place of the other. Perhaps there are things worse than alcoholism, and when you take away alcohol from some patients, you've got to be pretty careful that you give him something important in its place, or he may kill himself. I do think that there is a considerable overlap with regard to how many patients are depressed and how many are alcoholic.

Dr. Usdin:

I recall that in one of my seemingly most successful "cures" of an alcoholic, the patient committed suicide when I was on a three day trip. I fear that this was a dramatic instance of curing the disease but killing the patient. In this particular instance, the patient was an individual with tremendous potential who was not functioning up to his full potential. He had certain psycho-sexual conflicts and a need occasionally to escape a haranguing wife. There is an axiom in psychiatry that possibly we do not heed sufficiently. The axiom is "Don't take away a defense unless the patient has something healthy or less unhealthy to substitute for it." The probability of a masked depression certainly entered in.

I have apprehension and misgivings when physicians too casually recommend that a person take a little toddy or tonic in the evening. Here I am especially thinking of patients in their late forties and fifties who may be having a latent depression and present a variety of symptoms—fatigue, disinterest, irritability and introversion. I think a certain number of these feel that the physician has given them license for drinking. This drinking can then get out of hand. Of course, you might say that they would have had something else if they had not become alcoholics. Would you comment on this, Dr. Solomon?

Dr. Solomon:

I think that there are some patients who benefit by having a drink recommended to them by their physician. Now, these are apt to be, in Boston, the Beacon Hill dowager type who regards liquor as coming from the devil and, therefore, to be shunned and avoided and they would not touch liquor unless you actually prescribed it as medicine. Then they take it, and enjoy it, and get benefit from it. Most people don't have to have such a prescription. But, as I say, there are exceptions and we do see them in Boston and in those instances I don't have any statistics as to how many of them become alcoholics. My hunch is that very few do.

Dr. Torre:

Alcohol seems to be a drug that relieves anxiety in many patients. However, many people who have obtained relief from anxiety by using alcohol as a tranquilizer will try it for symptoms other than anxiety. For example, when they become depressed, they will treat their depression with alcohol because they've learned that it does relieve anxiety. Alcohol is a poor anti-depressant drug, and very frequently, makes the depression worse rather than better. One of the major problems in the depressed patient who is using alcohol is diagnosis. I agree that the history that Dr. Knight was talking about earlier today is very important. Let me illustrate: the other day I saw a seventy-two-year-old president of a company who was dragged in by the vice-president, who said, "My boss is an alcoholic. Please hospitalize him for me." A careful history revealed that he had been drinking excessively only since he was sixty-nine years old. However, the physicians treating him felt that he was an alcoholic and he'd been treated as an alcoholic for over two years. From a careful history, it was very clear that before the age of sixty-nine, this man was not an alcoholic—he used alcohol quite judiciously and successfully. A person who successfully uses alcohol this long is not likely to become an alcoholic at sixty-nine. Further careful history taking revealed that this man was treating a rather severe depression with alcohol. As long as treatment was directed only to the alcoholism, the depression remained. As soon as I treated the depression and the depression cleared up, excessive use of alcohol disappeared.

Dr. Knight:

I was very interested in Dr. Solomon's recommendations regarding the treatment approach to the alcoholic, which I think are very good. The extensive and careful detailed physical examination, attention to sociological factors, working with people in the family and the community is, I am sure, the enlightened and most effective way of approaching such patients, but I wonder how many medical practitioners can do this. Is it practical, since I emphasized so much in my own discussion the exigencies of time which press the medical practitioner? I wonder if the answer is to be working on only a few alcoholics at a time. Perhaps the medical practitioner, if he has to use this amount of time and energy, may have to limit his intervention to one or a few. Perhaps adequate and thorough treatment of alcoholics is not practical outside of a clinic. I would like to hear from the audience.

Audience:

I'd like to ask, can psychiatrists do much for alcoholism? I've been very disappointed in getting help from psychiatrists for alcoholics. I have an alcoholic who has been committed to our state institution two or three times. They keep him there and he gets sobered up and, after about a month or two, send him back home and I still have to contend with him.

Dr. Solomon:

I could respond to that by saying that psychiatrists do have pretty good luck treating alcoholics. They cure a third of them, get a third of them a little better, and have no effect on the other third. These are exactly the same statistics that I think you can find in any alcoholic clinic, be it a medical directed alcohol clinic, psychiatric, or psychoanalytic. The figures seem strangely about the same. There will be failures, but then you have a lot of failures in internal medicine, too. What do you do for your arteriosclerotics and your chronic arthritics? By no means must you feel that we are trying to oversell psychiatry. There are plenty of failures in our field, and if you try to emulate our work, you'll have failures, as well. I have experience at Boston City Hospital with a number of alcoholics which we call "super alcoholics." Ethyl alcohol is too tame for them, so they go in for some of the higher alcohols—butyl, isopropyl alcohol, methyl alcohol—they just barely manage not to kill themselves with it. We see them, of course, when they don't kill themselves. The coroner sees them when they do. But we have quite a number of these. Some of them are addicted to paraldehyde, some to other drugs that they use and find successful substitutes.

Audience:

I would like to supplement what Dr. Usdin said relating to the vegetative symptoms of depression.

Years ago, Dr. Henry L. Bockus of Philadelphia, the Dean of Gastroenterology, pointed out three additional symptoms which I have confirmed are very important. The first is that, in addition to anorexia, many depressed people lose the ability to differentiate the taste of food. They'll tell you that all food tastes alike. In addition to this, many of them will complain of a bitter taste of food. The other contribution that he made is in calling attention to the frequency with which pyrosis, heartburn, is a symptom of masked depression. People with heartburn don't turn out to have gall bladder disease. They frequently are depressed. I would also like to supplement the list of symptoms by one question from the Cornell Index which I have felt was very helpful. The patient will come in smiling—the first visit—and the Index will ask them, "Do you often wish you were dead and away from it all?" The smile will vanish and out will pour the story underneath.

It is also interesting, relating to Dr. Solomon, that there are masked depressions in the obese. He mentioned the alcoholic. There was an article recently reporting a group from the army. In practice, we find this very frequently.

May I add one or two other indications of masked depression. Pain, which is not related to any organic source, particularly abdominal pain or severe back pain, can be an indication of a masked depression. Other forms of aberrant behavior, like gambling, and younger people running away from home, forms of delinquency, are also indications of masked depression. I imagine the list could be almost indefinitely prolonged. Would you agree, Dr. Usdin?

Dr. Usdin:

I fully agree with you. I would like to emphasize the factor of motivation of the alcoholic. Very often the alcoholic comes in and says 'I am here only because my wife insisted that I come." It is surprising how often a patient uses this tactic when he, himself, really wants to get help. But the wife and others have played in with the tactic, so like a child, he is begrudgingly coming in. He has a clay pigeon into which he can constantly stick his barbs. Initially, I establish my position with the patient that "I am very willing and interested in helping you but when *you* are ready to come back on your own because *you* want help, please call my secretary to make an appointment." The majority of these patients will come back and say "Well, Doctor, now I'd like to see you." The therapeutic relationship has then been properly established.

I feel a little more optimistic about treating alcoholics than Dr. Solomon has expressed himself. I wonder if he was speaking of a survey of psychiatrists as a whole or medical clinics as a whole. I believe that those physicians who have a little added interest or, let us say, whose personalities fit in comfortably therapeutically with the alcoholic patient get much better results than those who do not. Physicians can have some delightful therapeutic experiences if they are willing to invest something of themselves in treating alcoholics. I would wager that Dr. Solomon's personal statistics are far better than one third arrested.

One of the things that I use as an adjunct is Antabuse®. First of all, it establishes the motivation of the patient—in a way, they commit themselves. I won't go into many of the ways Antabuse can work at this time, but when we speak of medical practitioners seeing patients with alcoholism and doing supportive therapy, Antabuse can be a valuable ally. Antabuse should be prescribed under a physician's direction, and the patient should be seen at regular intervals even if but for a few minutes. There is a relationship going on. With this as an ally, I think many of you can do the type of therapy that would take some of the burden off our shoulders.

I'd like Dr. Knight to comment on what analysis can provide.

Dr. Knight:

About the only thing in common that psychoanalysis and, I think, the good old fashioned general practice of medicine might have, the only thing they share when well done, is an attempt at a level-headed, realistic minimizing of therapeutic zeal. By this I mean that we have come to understand that the urgent desire to get somebody over some kind of sickness and cure him and make him "happy ever after" is an impediment to treatment, especially in psychoanalysis. One can only proceed at the pace that the patient is able to work. One has to recognize fully the processes of growth that are inherent in him and work accordingly. I think this is not too different from what I understand to be the traditional attitude of a general practitioner in treating chronic illness. Dr. Solomon has mentioned that we must face the fact that there are physical disabilities that can't be cured. Well, I think the same is true with psychological disabilities. One goes along with these patients through the years. One establishes an effective relationship. One offers opportunities for help, when help is needed, and doesn't feel disappointed and defeated when a cure can't be effected. It seems to me that this is one of the most effective forms of psychotherapy. We in psychiatry have been a little guilty of introducing the theme that unhappy people, mildly depressed people, alcoholic people, or what have you, ought to be grasped, have something done to them, and then they become different people. You don't do this with most of your patients in general practice—you establish a relationship that exists through the years, you tide them over their various crises, their physical illnesses, and all their emotional disturbances that occur intermittently. But, in the long run, when an opportunity for growth is presented, you are there. You stay with them. You help the patient cope with the inevitable pains and disasters that are inherent in life.

I think that this type of approach, with the emphasis not so much on "I must cure this alcoholic or depressive person" but "I must stay with him—I must see to it that we have a clear, understandable contract with one another." I must, as Dr. Solomon pointed out, take a great interest in his physical make-up, with details of every little illness in it and, as much as time allows, his emotional and psychological existence. This is best suited for the medical practitioner. If this approach is followed, then periodically occasions will emerge in the course of a patient's life when, with help, he can take a leap forward, when he can put some things together and grow. We get into most of our trouble, in short, when we decide we are going to cure this person of what amounts to not so much an illness, but a whole disturbed existence, a whole disturbed way of experiencing his life. We do our most effective work when we step back and try to be a professional friend, consultant, colleague and assistant to this patient.

Dr. Solomon:

I am also a psychoanalyst. But before that, I am a psychiatrist, and before that, I am a neurologist, and before that, I am a physician, and before that, I'd like to think I am a scientist. There are things before those too, but I need not go into them. The fact is that the selection factor is so important in the statistical evaluation of the treatment of alcoholics. In our alcohol clinic at Boston City Hospital so many of our patients come from skid row. These are people who have lost almost all contact with family life and with ordinary civilized living. They have been alcoholics for many years, and they are very difficult to work with. We think we do pretty well that we are able to relieve a third of them. In my private practice, where much of my work is psychoanalytic, I also have a select group of very difficult alcoholics who have been through a lot of other doctoring before they reach me, and there, instead of getting one third better, I finally succeed in getting about 33⅓ per cent better.

Audience:

Does the panel think that the cured alcoholic can ever go back to social drinking?

Dr. Solomon:

I think the answer is yes. There have been a couple of controlled and well documented studies indicating that this is possible. However, I think it is very rare. As a general rule, it is better to take the stand that an alcoholic should never drink at all. He should avoid the first drink. Some of them say, "How about starting with the second?" But I do think that, as a working rule, you should try to establish that the alcoholic must not drink at all. I do think the exceptions are individuals who can be followed for long periods of time intensively in a kind of psychotherapeutic relationship which you have some confidence in. I have had some alcoholics who have been relieved of alcoholism as a real source of illness and have been able to use alcohol socially with benefit and without danger. This is rare.

Dr. Usdin:

I would like to second Dr. Solomon's comments and say that it is so scarce and so rare, that we ought to keep it a medical secret because too many persons will therefore attempt it. If they feel that one out of 200 can socially drink, they are convinced they are that one. I have had a couple of these cures to the extent that they have returned to drinking socially for several years, but let's keep it within the confines of the profession. Nearly every arrested alcoholic carries within him the hope that he can return to social drinking. Statistics prove the physician should do nothing to encourage this belief.

Dr. Knight:

We are talking today mainly about general practitioners. The outstanding difference between that which the general practitioner offers and that which all the specialists offer, including psychiatrists, is that the former establishes a relationship with a patient, which theoretically and ideally should exist for the rest of the patient's life and for the physician's life. He does not set up a relationship with the person simply for the purpose of curing X illness, Y illness or Z illness, although in the course of this relationship such illnesses will occur. He establishes a total patient-physician relationship which is the basic psychotherapeutic instrument. How he uses this will by its nature be different than the approach of the specialist. I am interested in hearing some opinions as to how this unending relationship can be evaluated as a factor in treatment. It is not the same kind of relationship that the psychotherapist establishes. As a psychiatrist, or analyst, or specialist of any sort, there is always the end point which must be reached when we decide that the patient has done, or not done, or never will get done, that which we set out to do. This is not so with the medical practitioner whose patient will theoretically and often actually be with him for his entire life. What does this factor mean in the treatment of alcoholism, depression or psychiatric conditions?

Dr. Usdin:

May I again emphasize that the patient with alcoholism has this as a neurotic symptom. As mentioned, it may be a substitute symptom, e.g., for depression. If you remove it, you do it mostly by substituting something else in its place.

Dr. Solomon:

Sometimes I have the feeling that when you substitute nonalcoholism it is just as severe a neurotic symptom as is alcoholism. With some of these Alcoholics Anonymous characters, you wonder if they were not better off when they were good solid alcoholics, because they can be so objectionable and obnoxious with their Alcoholics Anonymous work. You wonder what kind of life they are leading when they become quite so sanctimonious about their nondrinking. Nevertheless, I think the point is that you have to substitute something for this alcoholism and you try to make it something reasonable and helpful to the individual and not just a form of Bernard McFaddin type of health and weight lifting and that type of exaggerated nonalcoholism.

Dr. Torre:

Would someone like to respond to Dr. Knight's question about the longitudinal relationship of the medical practitioner to the patient? Can we have some general questions?

Audience:

The well-motivated alcoholic is not much of a problem. If they really want to quit drinking, I have had excellent results with Alcoholics Anonymous. The one that bothers me is the housewife who drinks only at home and makes life very miserable for her family, maybe socially prominent and well-accepted in public. You try to get in on a situation like that. They'll deny alcoholism. They'll say, 'Oh, I take a drink once in a while to help me go to sleep" or something like that, if they admit anything and it is practically impossible to get anything done for them. I wonder if there are any little secrets or tricks that can be used to help in a situation of that type.

Dr. Solomon:

In my opinion, these are among the most difficult cases in medicine or psychiatry. In housewives of this sort, the alcoholism serves some deep-going unconscious need and it is useless to work with them on a superficial basis. These are individuals who really need deep-going, prolonged, intensive, and, in my opinion, psychoanalytically oriented psychotherapy. I think Dr. Knight and Dr. Usdin would probably agree with this. Don't feel in such a case that you can get early beneficial results. There are all kinds of difficulties in this type of case, and it takes many months, sometimes years of prolonged therapy before they can be helped. However, some of them can be helped.

Audience:

Dr. Solomon, I think you have not yet answered one part of the question. How does the general physician motivate this housewife to get on the couch of the psychiatrist?

Dr. Solomon:

That is the disease—the fact that they don't really want to get over their alcoholism. They may say they do, but do not really want to. How to get them to go to a psychiarist is a problem that you face with many other kinds of disorders in your practice. If you have their confidence, you sit down and have a long talk with them. Take a full hour and then say that you feel that they would benefit by going over this more fully with a psychiatrist, pointing out that the psychiatrist nowadays is not just for mental cases, but also for emotional cases. I like to say there are three kinds of illnesses—physical, mental and emotional. I separate the emotional ones like this because they think, "Oh well, then mine is not mental after all." They don't mind so much being referred for emotional disturbances. Then maybe they will go.

Audience:

I always hope that they will make a mistake sometime. I have one such patient who is a wife of a rather prominent engineer in a plant. She finally made the mistake of driving her car while she was very intoxicated. She was picked up by the police, and this so embarrassed her that she went to her pastor who straightened her out. That is the only one of these I have ever had any success with. Another one went to a psychiatrist for about two years and resisted admitting to him that she was an alcoholic. About all she came out with was the conclusion that her husband was an S.O.B. and the psychiatrist was trying to help her learn to live with him.

Dr. Knight:

May I make a comment about this type of person? It is a very serious and disturbing type of problem. At the risk of sounding dramatic, I'd like to say that in my experience whenever such a patient appears, I have found that somebody in the family wants them dead. It has happened too often to be a coincidence that in the admittedly few cases of this sort that I have seen, they are, almost invariably, responding to either the husband or parent or someone's hostility, which produces self destructive reactions so that they proceed to drink themselves to death and refuse resolutely to do anything about it. There is an element of defensive hostility and revenge involved in their behavior. In this connection, on the rare occasions when I think some effective intervention has been mobilized, it was only through initial contact with the crucial relative, the compulsive diligent husband who insists that the best be done for his wife and also insists that the problem is insoluble. Looking for the destructive ingredients in the picture and working with the trouble in the environment of this patient is a means of trying to get her, eventually, to come in for individual treatment.

Dr. Solomon:

Do you feel that family therapy would be indicated in this kind of problem?

Dr. Knight:

That is the only approach I've seen that works.

Dr. Solomon:

I think you are right.

Dr. Usdin:

I would strongly agree with Drs. Knight and Solomon and would like to add that, as many alcoholic patients are resolving some of their conflicts, the upset of the status quo of their relationship may cause an exacerbation of anxiety of the patient's mate and then be productive of destructive techniques on the part of this mate. It may behoove the physician to alert the patient to early signs of this activity. The alcoholic often has married somebody below his or her socioeconomic or intellectual status, and the mate of the alcoholic patient might handle her or his feelings of insecurity by emphasizing the fact of how helpless and inadequate the alcoholic mate is. It is for this reason that counselling or therapy of the mate or relative with whom the patient lives is indicated.

Audience:

I'd like to ask the panel about how well qualified a psychologist is to aid in treating depression. I've always used psychologists to test or evaluate, particularly the intellect of a child and so forth. I have a colleague who has referred a child about thirteen years old who is quite depressed—wouldn't go to school and so forth—to this psychologist and he has seen the child five or six times and the father eight or ten times. He has given me a report since I have taken over the child. I just wonder how much weight to put on this report and if he is qualified to treat this child.

Dr. Knight:

You touch on an area which is of considerable concern to the field of psychiatry—that is, its relationship to psychology. As far as I am concerned, personally, no nonmedical person can assume total responsibility for the treatment of a patient. However well-trained a psychologist may be, they must function in a setting which allows for medical scrutiny. Medical collaboration or medical supervision of one sort or another is mandatory. We must readily acknowledge that the training of many psychologists is quite adequate The therapy they perform is in many instances not too different than that of a medical psychotherapist. My only reservation is that one can't assume responsibility for a person sick in one area, unless one has at least been trained so that he may be able to pick up disturbances in other areas of functioning, and this can only be done by a physician. So, I would say if your consulting psychologist is functioning in a setting where medical supervision is available to him, then you could have confidence in him.

Audience:

You mean nonpsychiatric?

Dr. Knight:

I mean psychiatric or nonpsychiatric. There must be a physician in a position to see what is going on in the treatment, such as is found in a clinic setting and perhaps in private collaboration.

Dr. Solomon:

May I add one comment. Not only should you be interested in the generic differences of the consultant, whether he is a psychiatrist or a psychologist, or a what not, but I think you should not overlook the importance of individual differences. I think you ought to keep in mind that you are entitled to make the choice and to discriminate between what you consider to be a good member of that particular professional specialty and what you consider to be one somewhat less than adequate.

Audience:

I wonder if there is not a time when you do condemn the person or the personality, occasionally not confining your condemnation to the alcoholism or apparent illness? So many alcoholics are dependent personalities, dependent people, and the general practitioner so often is the father image type of person or respected person that occasionally not only gives support but also firm direction. It has proven effective to jump on their bottoms a little bit, to reprimand them personally. I'd like to have your opinion on that, and also on the treatment of alcoholics. The physician from Georgia made a comment about the number of alcoholics who would turn up at the state hospital where they were just washed out and sobered up. This seems like a fine opportunity to get psychiatric consultation which we don't have. The same thing apparently accomplishes what we accomplish when we see one for the first time. Any physician can usually handle an acute phase, dry them out, prevent some deliriums, and what not. However, I think there is some deficiency in some of the state institutions in giving consultation to a medical practitioner, and helping him in long term treatment.

Dr. Knight:

Your comment about one's reactions to difficult patients is

interesting to me. Part of my urging you to make notations of behavior and emotions includes the assumption on my part that one's own reactions can occasionally be included in these notations. This, I think, is important. Some years ago, Dr. Karl Menninger, in writing up an outline for psychiatric history-taking, recommended a section at the beginning for subjective reactions, in effect saying, "Put down your real reactions to this person—whether you like him or don't like him and why. After you have gotten all this down, then you can at least try to be a little objective in the remainder of the examination." I think that there is some merit in the business of fully facing your feelings about a patient. I won't go into any further detail than to say that if one is really irritated and angry at a patient, one should never attempt to undertake the responsibility of psychotherapy. On the other hand, there is always something in every patient that may be worked with. I recall an old Jewish proverb which states that if you search long enough and hard enough, in the heart of every man you will find somewhere a poem. This has sustained me through literally years of pursuit, in the assumption that there somewhere must be something creative or unique about each person, however hopeless the case may seem at the time. I hesitate to think that the medical practitioner would have to sustain himself solely on this basis. It is perhaps a point that depends on your philosophic viewpoint.

Dr. Solomon:

I would endorse what Dr. Knight has just said, but in further answer to the questioner, I would say this: you may be getting good results from taking a severe condemnatory attitude under certain circumstances with certain individuals, but I don't think it is because you've condemned it. I think it is because you showed him how sincere you were in wanting to help him. In other words, I think it is a by-product of that that's made him realize that you really are concerned about him, that you really want to get him better. If you show it in this particular way, that isn't so terribly important. I do agree with you that it's terribly important to let a person realize that you are sincere and that you feel strongly about what you are telling him. However, I stand by my guns that it is better not to condemn him. Condemn what he has done, and you don't really have to put much emphasis on it. He knows it is wrong. Everybody has been telling him that forever, and he knows it in his own heart. Show your sincerity in some other way.

Now what I've just said is just as applicable to bringing up children. You must show sincere desire to help them, for their sake. This is what the good parent does. You condemn their mistakes, you don't condemn the child. But even if you do condemn the child and the child feels you are doing it for his sake, the mistake doesn't make too much difference. You can be the kind of parent who wallops the kid once in a while, or you can be the kind who sends him to his room, and so on. It isn't so much the method, it's what's behind it that counts. If you really are trying to prove to that patient how much you want to get him better, this is going to sustain him and be of therapeutic value even if you do it in your own particular way or some other way. One last comment. I am reminded of when I went to medical school which was a long time ago. We had just gotten over a state of affairs in the treatment of diphtheria in which the textbooks gave actually fifty different recommendations on how diphtheria should be treated. You know, "This is apt to be good under some circumstances, or you may try that, or many people feel this is desirable." They went through all these different treatments for diphtheria and just then diphtheria antitoxin came up. You never hear a word about any of those fifty methods any more because now we know how to treat diphtheria scientifically. So what I want to say about the treatment of alcoholism is that we've got lots of methods, and this is good and that's good and they're all just wonderful. I have a feeling that it won't be long before we will find something scientifically far more valuable and then we will have a much better chance to get the results we all want.

Dr. Usdin:

I think Dr. Knight, with his "looking for the poem," Dr. Solomon, with his taking the patient as a whole emphasized the Gestalt theory which was what I was trying to say when I was talking about depressive reactions. Look at the whole person, because very often the patient is looking at an unfortunate part of himself or his situation and is fixated on that point. This usually is not the basic cause of the depression—it can be the focus.

We can tie up these subjects. Dr. Knight spoke of the homicidal actions of a family; sometimes when the woman is an alcoholic, one can see that the family is trying to kill her. We can think of alcoholism often being a suicidal thing on the part of the patient. We have masked suicides as well as masked depressions. We also have alcoholics who have no overt suicidal, intent driving cars in a manner that may be very suicidal, and there are a large number of accidents that are happening unconsciously or, again, with alcoholism. So, a lot of this ties in with what we've been talking about this morning.

ADOLESCENTS—DISTURBED AND DISTURBING

JOHN P. LAMBERT, M.D.

IN TALKING ABOUT the adolescent, I am reminded of the weather, "Everybody talks about it but there's not much you can do about it." "If you don't like the way it is, just wait a little while and it will change." Adolescence has been described as a "Disorder of time, cured by the passage of time"; yet as one perceptive adolescent remarked, "some never get into adolescence and others never get out of it." At any rate, we have all been adolescent and survived. Currently there are a tremendous number of persons (what with nearly half the population under twenty-five) who are in that stage between the child and the adult, at least chronologically; many are disturbing and disturbed. This holds true also for the family and the setting in which they live. I have nothing to offer that is new or original, no pill, prescription or cook book recipe to be taken or dispensed by the medical practitioner who is seeing an increasing number of problems in terms of the adolescent and his family. There are, however, some points that can be made which may be useful to the physician and may make it easier for him to help the teenager and the parents. Those points which will be discussed deal with the following.

1. An orientation or way of looking at the adolescent, each parent, and the situations in which they are involved.
2. The recognition and understanding of the struggles taking place in and among members of a family.
3. The doctor's role and contribution to better individual and family adjustment.

It is easily seen that the adolescent and his family are often

114

disturbed within themselves as well as disturbing to each other. The father, mother, and child are out of step. Each pleads, or even demands, that the other get in step. The parent is the one who usually comes to the medical practitioner. A wide range of attitudes and behavior of the teenager may be described by the troubled parent who is often confused, frightened, hurt, and even angry. Let us look at some examples:

> A college freshman spent time visiting cafes near the water-front talking with sailors, was nearly arrested, and said, "I was just wanting to live." Jim wanted to stay up all night "to see what it feels like." Jane wanted to "go with a boy I don't trust or like because I want to have experience." Pete wears his hair long with sideburns, boasts of his masculinity and seems to be unaware that his hair style makes him look like a girl. Sue, who "will talk for hours on the telephone but only utter mono-syllables" to her parents, "is always a mess with no sense of what to wear," yet criticized her mother's lack of stylishness. A fifteen year old whose parents said, "we can't cope with his rebellious and hostile behavior." Joe won't go to school and wants to go out at night wtih a bum group. He sneaks out the window and has stayed out all night.

Such situations are complicated and are both a challenge and a threat to the physician. However, in providing health care over a period of time to a family, the medical practitioner is in a unique and sensitive position to make significant contributions to individual and family adjustment. The medical practitioner is in a somewhat different position than the psychiatrist, in that he is usually known by the family and has some preexisting relationship with them. Many times families find it difficult to bare some of the problems to a person they know and prefer a stranger. It is difficult for the physician too. There are certain points that can be made that may facilitate recognition and understanding of what's going on and what can be done about it. The first of these is an awareness of one's own *role* as well as those thrust upon one. (Though it may be artificial, the physician may take the position, "let us assume for the moment that we have never met and know nothing of each other.") In this way one may get a clearer overall picture. Confronted by an angry

mother and her frightened sixteen-year-old daughter Mary, who
has missed her period, how does he feel? What does he do?
What if he has a teenage son or daughter?

Most persons, even the professional, initially get caught up
emotionally under such circumstances. It is imperative for the
physician, if he is to be helpful, to be able to be objective and
somewhat detached though not aloof or remote. His own
biography, past or present, his own anxieties, fears, and prejudices
should be kept out of the situation in which he is currently
involved. Above all, he must be accepting and understanding,
and at all times remember his professional role. He must be alert
to certain types of parent. They may try to take him out of his
professional role. We all know some of these types: the *socializing*
or *fraternizing* one who wants to be palsy-walsy, and says, "You
and I together will take care of this situation"; the *deferential*
one who in effect says, "Yes, father," and dumps all the responsibility in your lap; there is the *dependent* one who is clinging,
wanting all sorts of advice, and resists all understanding; then
there is the *self-blaming* one who speaks of all his (or her) sins
of omission and commission, who is basically trying to "take
credit" for all of the patient's difficulties; lastly, there is the
mechanical one, the robot, who goes by the book and authorities,
has all the words but no music. Despite the type, I want to
emphasize that each parent basically wishes and is trying to be a
good father or mother.

The physician must be an authority without being authoritarian. He must maintain his professional role. If he does not,
and sides with either parent, child, or attempts to be a referee
between them, there is one inevitable consequence. He is caught
up in a power struggle in which he is bound to lose to the
detriment of all concerned. He has joined the parents and child
in a revolving door where it is hard to know who is chasing
whom and who is running from whom.

The physician is more likely to be objective and have a sense
of perspective if he is able to recognize and understand what is
going on in the adolescent, in the parent, and the interactions
between them—adolescent, mother, and father. This calls for a
somewhat different orientation or point of view than is cus-

tomarily held by the medical practitioner. By tradition, training and daily medical practices, he focuses usually on the individual, his symptoms, organs and systems. In dealing with the adolescent and his family, it is useful to look at the total family as a unit, with its various individual parts interacting and influencing each other. In addition, he must include the past and present socio-cultural setting. The physician must accept in principle, if not recognize, that each one, parent as well as child, is within himself having a struggle. Besides this internal, personal, individual struggle, there is a struggle between and among members of the family, and thirdly, there is a struggle between the family and other families (society). While each of these struggles may differ outwardly in its form or content, they have in common a basic goal—survival-safety-security. Behavior must be looked upon as a security measure, though what makes one secure, may make another insecure. To illustrate: A headmaster was quite disturbed over the "definance of authority" of a fourteen-year-old boy in lighting up a cigarette in his office, which led to expulsion. Jim had been sent away to Boarding School to remove him from a broken home situation. The boy had brought about his return home through breaking a rule flagrantly.

The essential elements of the struggle within the adolescent and his rebellion against the parents are pretty well known by everybody. It is important for one to remember to see behavior in young people as a way of dealing with anxieties arising from their mixed feelings of dependency and independency and developing sexual urges. It is one thing to recognize these principles and quite another to apply them in the face of the dramatic attempts on the part of the adolescent to throw off parental controls and seeks to establish his own sense of status and identity. The adolescent tends to devalue and belittle the parent. It seems as if the adolescent must take this step to make progress toward adult status. The devaluations are apt to involve parental ideas, ideals, and ways of living. Belittlement comes in the criticism of parent's clothing, the home, or of almost anything. The adolescent may become extremely critical of the parents' social and political philosophies and take perverse delight in puncturing the most idealistic notions of their parents. This devaluation is most difficult for parents to meet with equanimity. It can best be understood as a part of the effort of an immature personality to win definition for itself.

Often there is associated with this devaluation of the parents a repudiation of the whole growing up process. There is an attempt to deny maturity or to postpone as long as possible taking over the responsibilities that biological maturation imposes. The dirty, disheveled, sloppy stage of early adolescence can be seen as a rebellion against the parents' earlier insistence on neatness and cleanliness. There is also implied in this almost studied lack of pride in personal appearance a way of denying any interest in what members of the opposite sex will think of them. The child is able to utilize this way of dressing to deny both parental training and adolescent growth. It is a part of the "I hate women" or "I'm never going to get married" stage. Some girls express the same repudiation of the feminine role with an active tomboyishness and interest in strenuous athletic activities, and in some extreme instances almost starving themselves to avoid the development of mature feminine bodily configurations.

Along with the active devaluation of the parent there begin to appear strong attachments on the part of adolescents to older men and women. The boy seeks out older men, teachers, club leaders, friends of the family and the like; girls seek out attachments to older women. There are strong desires to emulate these people. When these attachments are made the opinions and ideas of these older people are accepted by the adolescent as infallible; they are worthwhile and valuable and more in accord with facts than are the ideas or opinions of the parents. Parents are quite likely to become frustrated when their child turns outside the home to other adults for guidance, especially when the shortcomings and deficiencies of these other adults are known to them.

The adolescent continues his devaluation of the parent and his struggle to disassociate himself from parental control in relation to school programs and vocational plans. He may believe that the school of his parents' choice is satisfactory but disagree violently about the course selected for him; it is too hard and will never be any use to him. There is a similar indecision and lack of acceptance of parental values around vocational choices. They may change from week to week with the advent of new teachers or new children in the neighborhood. The adolescent will not permit himself to accept the parents' ideas.

Another aspect of parent devaluation is seen in the quiet secretive child who looks for confirmation or denial of his ideas or opinions to someone outside the home. The friend of the same age is able to give estimates of values and has a knowledge of things far superior to that of any adult, especially the parent. Questions addressed to the child about prosaic matters of day to day living receive no answer or at best, a grunt. An attitude of resigned tolerance meets the parents' concern over what the boy or girl might be doing.

During midadolescence, as a rule the youngster's desire to be a part of a group becomes imperative. In his drive for emancipation and achievement of independency of action he turns to the group of people his own age to support and reassure him in his independence from home. The group helps him in his physical and emotional breaking away from the home. The trend is to a strong conformity to the group patterns, to group needs, even though the behavior that results is condemned by adults and parents. It is to be remembered: that even though the conspicuous aspects of adolescent group behavior do not correspond to the usual adult standards, the adolescent group behavior does represent attempts to anticipate and understand adult status. The tolerance the adolescent develops to adult disapproval and restraint is an important part of his attempt to secure and maintain ultimate independent adult status. Acceptance by the group may seem, to the parent, more important than acceptance by the parent. Most adolescents, however, are somewhat torn in their attempts to satisfy the standards of a group and that of the parents. For the dependent adolescent or conscientious one the double orientation may be very disturbing; it makes him feel guilty and resentful and promotes anxiety.

Adolescents are in need of group acceptance. They become uncomfortable if they are in any way considered out of step or peculiar. The group will have its fad of dress and personal appearance. The particular clothes or the manner of wearing the hair (so disturbing to parents) is the adolescent's way of gaining security by belonging to the group as he is trying to emancipate from the parents. Many adolescents are concerned about some physical difficulty. They are too fat or too thin, too tall or too short. They may show undue concern over skin blemishes, body odors, or some barely noticeable defect. They may attribute their lack of success in the social group to the defect, whereas the lack of social success is the cause for the dissatisfaction with appearance.

In these various aspects of the adolescent drive for independence and emancipation the alternating phases of a need for independence and a need for dependence can be seen. The adolescent is unable to give up his childhood dependency completely nor can he refuse to grow up. In adolescence the child does not feel capable of controlling his needs and destinies completely, even though at times his apparent rebellion against parental authority may seem to indicate the opposite. Parents and other adults who deal with the adolescent need to be quite tolerant of the conflicts and behavior of the period. If the aggressive repudiation of the parent elicits an aggressive response on the part of the parent a vicious cycle is immediately set up. An impasse results from which neither the child nor the parent can retreat without considerable loss of face. At times the rebellion against unreasonable and harsh parental authority may spread to all other established rules of living in school and in the community. By and large, the adolescent is unhappy about the rebellion inherent in his drive for emancipation and adult status; the hostility he feels toward those who interfere with his blundering attempts to grow up may lead to guilt feelings and anxiety. Most children, however, are able to emancipate themselves without serious or long lasting upset. The child whose adjustments in infancy and childhood have been satisfactory is in the best position to meet this first problem peculiar to the adolescent period without undue stress or strain.

The second of the developmental tasks of adolescence is concerned with those problems centering around the *control and sublimation* of the sexual instinct. It is no longer assumed that the sexual interests and activities appear for the first time at puberty at the time of physiological maturation of the reproductive system. From his earliest days the child has been forced by parental attitude and social pressures to establish controls in relation to the purely physiological and anatomical aspects of the sexual drive and the expression of the associated various bodily pleasures. Only partial expressions of these drives have been permitted. The diffuse, varied and only partially developed components of the sexual drive in childhood are to be distinguished from the more complex, unified, mature form of the sexual instinct as it appears in adolescence. In adolescence the objective of the sexual instinct becomes the biological function of reproduction. There is a biological intensification of sexual urges at puberty. The controls established earlier in life may well no longer be adequate when the strong heterosexual drive emerges in adolescence. In the normal course of personality maturation, the adolescent has to establish certain controls of these inner drives in the process of accepting sexuality as an important part of the personality and adjusting to it. In most instances, this is accomplished without too much difficulty. Some adolescents, however, because of inadequate or too rigid training in early childhood in other spheres as well as sexual matters, may establish defenses against sexual expression which may be so severe and extreme as to be quite disabling. These individuals may not be able to face in themselves any of the evidences of sexual impulse or urges which are commonly found in adolescence, sexual phantasies, urges toward association with members of the opposite sex, urges for masturbation and the like.

The ways in which the controls are established in the young child and become changed in the adolescent may be summarized (after Gitelson) briefly. In early childhood, parental authority is apt to be accepted as a definite external reality. This derives out of the child's dependence on the parents and emotional attachment to them. The more satisfactory the parent-child relationships are the more easily this authority becomes established as an internal psychic factor which helps the child in the management of his underlying urges and drives. In the adolescent the strivings for emancipation and independency, in the course of which rebellion against parental authority takes place, over-reach their developmental purpose and alienate the child from these internalized representations of parental control and parental example. This leaves the adolescent largely on his own, psychically. Most of the contradictory and inconsistent aspects of adolescent emotional life seem to be manifestations of a precarious balance maintained between the controls and defenses utilized by the adolescent and the powerful underlying psychological and biological drives which become exacerbations at puberty. The characteristic emotional life of the adolescent has been well described by Anna Freud. "Adolescents are excessively egoistic, regarding themselves as the center of the universe and the sole object of interest, and yet at no time in later life are they capable of so much self-sacrifice and devotion. They form the most passionate love-relationships only to break them off as abruptly as they began them. On the one hand they throw themselves enthusiastically into the life of the community and, on the other, they have an over powering longing for solitude. They oscillate between blind submission to some self-chosen leader and defiant rebellion against any and every authority. They are selfish and materially minded and at the same time full of lofty idealism. They are ascetic but will suddenly plunge into instinctual indulgence of the most primitive character. At times their behavior to other people is rough and inconsiderate, yet they themselves are extremely touchy. Their moods veer between lighthearted optimism and the blackest pessimism. Sometimes they will work with indefatigable enthusiasm and at other times they are sluggish and apathetic."

Some adolescents need, in order to protect themselves from the overwhelming anxieties attendant to the increase in and change in the direction of the sexual drives, to develop defenses or methods of control which in themselves may be disabling.

One example of an extreme defense are tendencies on the part of the adolescent to periods of marked shyness and withdrawal. These may involve so great a part of his daily life to make those about him concerned as to his mental health. Usually, however, this is a defensive phase through which the child goes as he builds up within himself more adequate controls which will permit him a normal response to his sexual drives.

Another kind of defense may be an over-reaction to the sexual feelings so that the adolescent assumes that anything to do with sexual strivings, or even anything to do with a member of the opposite sex is necessarily bad and sinful. This asceticism may spread to include among the activities in which the adolescent will not participate—anything pleasurable, attractive clothing, music, movies, dancing. Others may deny themselves protection against cold, reduce daily food intake to a minimum, force themselves to get up early, arrange rigorous physical exercise programs, and in extreme instances, defer defecation or urination as long as possible, rationalizing this as not giving in to one's physical needs. Clinically at times we observe such behavior as a reaction to guilt over adolescent masturbation and gross sexual phantasies.

Another defense which at times may be extreme is observed, usually in later adolescence. The individual may turn to endless intellectualizations of his problems. He may become preoccupied with some new radical or even ultraconservative type of social order. He becomes preoccupied with abstractions and likes to talk about them with the friends he forms. The variety of problems which he may discuss is great. Is life worth living? Has it a purpose? Has it a meaning? Is idealism worth while? etc. The solutions he constructs for various real and alleged social and economic problems he believes to be realistic. The solutions he finds make little difference in his actual behavior. The intellectual discussions are not bone fide attempts at solving reality problems. Basically they are attempts at solving his own emotional conflict about the expression of his own individual needs and desires in the society in which he finds himself.

A final type of defense may be mentioned. This is the adolescent's tendency to form transient relationships with others. These apparently intensely emotional attachments to other persons, both their contemporaries and older individuals, are not meaningful interpersonal relationships, as occur in maturity. The adolescent, through a process of identification, borrows in a magical way the strengths of those who appear to be strong. This borrowing is done in an undiscriminating way and without assimilating. The apparent fickleness of the adolescent is a result of his constant search for some way of protecting himself from the internal forces which are disturbing him. For a time he is able to get some measure of comfort and support by taking over some of the characteristics of the friend of the moment. As the model changes one can often recognize who is the friend he admires. The adolescent may take over the methods of dress, handwriting, personal mannerisms, as well as the social, political and other views. These change as the friendship is abandoned and another one takes its place.

It is important for those who deal wtih adolescents, parents and others, to recognize these defenses for what they are, and if necessary, to try to help the child. They are, no matter how unsatisfactory, the best defenses he can establish at the time, to control the urgency of his drive and to protect himself from the emotional discomfort which arises. It is indicated in the discussion above that some of the defenses may become so extreme as to become socially disabling to the adolescent. It is, in the words of the old saw, a situation where the cure may be worse than the disease. By and large, the adolescent who has not developed in his earlier childhood a sense of security, who has not prior to his teenage been able to develop ways of managing and counteracting his strong internal drives, whose relationships with his parents have not provided the necessary emotional support and direction that he needs for satisfactory progress in his journey to emotional maturity, is the one whose defenses become disabling. The secure, well adjusted child will proceed through the emotionally turbulent adolescent years with a minimal disturbance to himself and others. He follows the characteristic trial and error path in his attempts to emancipate himself and in learning to accept his sexuality and to adjust to it. His responses do not, however, reach the extreme degrees which prevent him from acknowledging his sexual drives and patterning them to what society demands. Nor do his strivings for emancipation prevent him from maintaining his family contacts and accepting his dependency status until the time comes for him to be an independent self-supporting and self sufficient adult.

The elements of the struggle within the parent are as important as those of the adolescent. Mother and father were once adolescents with problems and parents. This has many implications for the parent as their child enters adolescence. It tends to reawaken old experiences and unsolved problems. The adult is disturbed by the changing status of its offspring and feels the loss of love which the change from dependency creates. Not infrequently, when the adolescent is asserting its independency, the parent will be pulling him back to a childhood status; when he feels the need to be dependent, the parents more often look for a young adult who will assume responsibilities. Parents, like adolescents, have mixed feelings of dependency and independency.

The reaction of the parent to the adolescent's behavior is determined not only by how the parent sees the teenager, but also by the parental needs to adapt to social and cultural forces. Does the parent unwittingly see the child as a part or extension of itself, an agent, a rival, or as a separate unique individual? I am sure you have all seen such situations as the parent with limited education wanting its child to go through college, the mother treating her daughter as a sister, the parent whose security in his social system is threatened by non-conforming behavior of the child. Thus, how the child fits into the parents' psychic economy determines the extent to which the parent's equanimity is disturbed. There are many instances in which the adolescent behavior is an expression of a parental desire or reenactment in principle of parental behavior. The parent may be more or less aware of such desires or wishes. The less acceptable such wishes are to the parent the more likely is he or she to over-react to the adolescent expression of them.

Then there is the struggle of the family with other families and social cultural values about which the same conflicts about dependency-independency arise. To illustrate, what happens when two adolescents of different religion and ethnic backgrounds start getting serious about marriage?

The physician, in his interested but objective position, can be very helpful and supporting to both the parent and the child. He must be able to see the meaning of the struggle and the meaning of the behavior before he is in a position to work with the individuals in helping them help themselves.

The physician's grasp and understanding of what is going on can be facilitated if he utilizes certain principles in his evaluation of the situation.

1. All the behavior has its roots in an attempt by the parent and the child to maintain or gain security in the face of change. The parent and child both have mixed feeling about this goal of reaching an adult status. It is a matter of checks and balances, actions and reactions. In each there is much uncertainty and doubt about changes, as the child is moving through adolescence toward an adult status.

2. The individual during adolescence must deal with two special problems: emancipation or separation from the family and a control and sublimation of the sexual drive.

3. The unsolved problems that a parent had with its parents tend to reappear with the spouse and are unwittingly imposed on the child.

4. No serious maladjustments arise in adolescence without significant disturbances having been present in earlier years.

Generally, one gets the story first from the parent when it concerns a young adolescent. Frequently, it has been found wiser, in the long run, to see an older adolescent before seeing the parent. Sometimes the parents and child are seen together. A joint session is helpful in seeing objectively some of the interactions in the parent-child relationships. One should get a separate story from each parent and the child. The physician must listen alertly to the story as it spontaneously unfolds. If the initial statements are recorded verbatim it is often surprising how, in the course of this, attitudes and feelings of the individual are often unwittingly revealed in side remarks and the way of phrasing an answer.

A mother says, "I don't know what I would do without my mother." Another, "It's funny I didn't have half the time to spend with my second child." A father speaking of his wife, "Mom and I are not displeased." A boy saying of his henpecked and milktoast father, "I am so afraid of my father's temper."

It is seldom that an account of the situation by the parent bears much resemblence to that given by the adolescent. Parents and children have different points of view. They see the world differently and each has difficulty in communicating with the other, but each can do so with an outsider they trust. The physician can fill this role but must not carry stories. It behoves the doctor to remember words are slippery things, people seldom say all they mean, nor mean all they say. He must tune in on the messages that are expressed indirectly. (Importance of this has been pointed out by previous speakers.) Such messages are usually for help and protection. They indicate a search for gratification of a craving for dependency. The adolescent, in his urge to be independent and self-reliant, finds it difficult to acknowledge or accept such dependency desires or, there may be no acceptable person available to whom he may turn or, aid is desired from some neutral and far removed authority.

Often, the "acting out" behavior which disturbs adults carries the message that there is too much or too little authority or structuring for the needs of the adolescent. Such acting out behavior may be an indication that the adolescent does not know where he stands, or that he has no place to move. We all like to know where we stand. We all depend upon the white line on the highway to guide us.

As the family physician collects and sorts the information given, his own observations of the moment as well as those he has accumulated over the years in various contacts with the family, he may find himself wondering. "Is this a sick adolescent—or is this an adolescent reacting to a sick situation—or just a transient growth disturbance?" Many times it is difficult to differentiate the approximate 10 per cent of pathologically sick from the "normative reactions." There are no isolated pathognomic criteria unless it be peer evaluation. The adolescent peer group is most sensitive to what is going on and quickly differentiates the "sick" from the disturbed and disturbing.

It can be said there are no significant disturbances in adolescence that have not had clear cut preceding maladjustment. One sees during adolescence wide swings of mood and interest, order and disorder behind which lies a number of processes and struggles interacting with each other. It is difficult to know just what is going on at any given moment. If one considers just the external life of the adolescent it can be quite misleading. The outward disorganized pattern is not always a reflection of an internal mental disorganization. At any given moment, the behavior of the adolescent may suggest a mental illness particularly if one looks at such characteristics as: the intensity and volatillity of their feelings, their inability to tolerate any anxiety, the demand for immediate gratification, poor reality testing, the lack of self-criticism, and tendency to see the world differently than the adult does. Most of these characteristics, unless in excessive quantity and carried on over a long period, are not pathologic. The physician should bear in mind the possibility of suicide by the adolescent. This may occur when the patient suffers the loss (death, destruction, defeat) of a person, object or goal in which he has a tremendous and real emotional investment. When there has been a large accumulation of resentment there may be impulsive spitefulness that ends in tragedy. The physician can be reassured in the main if the child is able to give an orderly account of his "special" behavior (in contrast to not speaking or acknowledging bizarre performance) and his peers do not see him as "sick." When there is prolonged withdrawal and preoccupation, extreme asceticism, and a history of impulse behavior that the child is unable to control or modify, special help should be sought.

As the physician is able to recognize and understand what is going on in the adolescent, in the parent, in the interaction between the adolescent and the parent, and has knowledge of the setting in which this is taking place, and an awareness of his own role and the roles thrust upon him, he is in a unique and strategic position to help in relation to the adolescent and his family. Such help can be direct and indirect by his attitude. He should have a genuine interest in the parent and the adolescent, have a respect of the uniqueness of the individuals and the differences between people. Above all have a willingness to listen, to try to understand and to be of help, i.e., to care, have the capacity to function as an authority without being authoritarian. He must not mix in his personal uncertainties, doubts and anxieties into those of the parent and teenager. He should be able to offer alternatives that permit a choice. It must be remembered that much of the fighting that goes on is not to win or lose but to have the freedom to choose. Both parent and child must be able to save face and not feel humiliated. The physician can help each person, to the extent that is appropriate and acceptable, see the meaning of the struggle and the meaning of the behavior. His tolerance and acceptance of things as they are is often supporting and may rub off on members of the family. He should be able to desensitize special issues and deflect feelings to less sensitive areas. It is important to encourage and give praise when due so that each will try again if one feels defeated. The basic goal of the physician is working with not on or for, the individuals to help them help themselves.

Most of what has been said can be summed up with a true clinical situation about which there are many implications for discussion.

Mrs. Russo, about forty-five, of Irish descent, brought her only child, Mary Ellen, a petit though fully mature twelve and a half year old to the Pediatric Clinic with a variety of complaints: "pains in the stomach that are terrible on weekends, won't pay attention to me, gets high fevers, doing poorly in school." The mother rather pevishly attributed the onset of difficulties to the menarche at ten years. She stated, "Maybe if she hadn't taken care of herself so soon, been so sorta on her own since she could walk, she wouldn't had her period so early and we'd not had those pains." There did not seem to be anything else unusual about Mary's development and adjustment.

Mary, somewhat sullen and shy, merely said, "I have terrible pains sometimes but it doesn't hurt now. I don't need an examination." The mother became quite angry at this. The medical student suggested to Mary that it wasn't necessary to get all undressed and he would do the examination later. He continued to write down the rambling story given by the mother who described a variety of somatic complaints experienced by her "like when I was pregnant" but which had not been incapacitating or led to much doctoring. Rather bitterly she told of becoming pregnant "because the church told me to—that it would make our marriage. I had wanted to leave my husband and now would except for that child."

Mrs. Russo played bingo several nights a week and had visited her father's grave every Sunday afternoon for fourteen years. "My husband just watches or listens to the ball game on Sunday afternoons—I hate baseball—it makes me so mad."

The medical student suggested that Mrs. Russo and her husband might talk, something they never did, about their troubles over what to do on Sundays and report back the following week.

Mrs. Russo returned, with a more friendly and open Mary saying, "she hasn't had the pains anymore." Mother continued with obvious pleasure—"My husband went to the cemetery with me on Sunday morning—Mary and I went to the movies in the afternoon while Carmen went to the ball park." The medical student, plainly delighted, was quite complimentary to the mother for what she had accomplished and asked for a follow up report. About three weeks later Mary and the parents returned. Mother and daughter seemed relaxed and pleasant with each other. Mary, seen alone, was full of questions about her feelings toward her parents, her concern about her size and social adjustment and about sex. She voiced concern over her ability to handle herself and indicated a need for an acceptance of an outside authority when she said with a smile, "I don't want to come back again but I know you won't let me get away not coming back."

Mr. Russo indicated there had been a change in his wife and rounded out the over all picture with, "She and her father were fighting all the time—he didn't want us to get married—I think he wanted her to just keep house for him. It doesn't make sense to go to the cemetery so often—she doesn't owe him anything and I am not going along with it every week."

Mrs. Russo stated, "Maybe he is stuck on baseball because I go to bingo—we have plans to take a trip in the country over next weekend."

COUNSELING WITH FAMILY PROBLEMS

IRWIN M. MARCUS, M.D.

T HE ROLE OF counselor for a patient and his family is not new in medical practice. This activity has always been included within the art of practicing medicine, along with physical procedures and medication aimed toward restoring and maintaining health. Just as scientific knowledge and skill have grown in the physical aspects of medicine, so has the understanding of the ingredients of the doctor-patient relationship expanded. The patient is seen not only as an individual interacting within his own total system, but also as one who is enmeshed in family interaction and in larger social forces. Individuals undergoing strong emotional reactions to family and other social pressures require early effective intervention before the effect of the stress results in serious mental or physical signs of decompensation or collapse.

Counseling is a form of psychotherapy and its effectiveness will depend upon the physician's grasp of the situation, his talent in communication, the timing of his intervention, and the appropriateness of the goals he is setting for his course of action. The ability of the physician to define the conflict and identify the sources of anxiety he perceives in the family varies with the level of self-understanding and family feeling he has achieved. His flexibility and empathy must be such as to avoid a rigid and prejudicial response which would only cloud and confuse the problem.

The concepts in family psychotherapy are still in an early phase of development and most of the studies on family psychopathology have lacked control groups. The type of problem or pathology present must determine the approach as is the case

131

in other aspects of medical practice. Family counseling may be done with the family as a group, or there may be circumstances for seeing the family members individually or in various combinations in a flexible manner.

In medical practice, we wouldn't attempt treatment without a diagnostic impression of the illness based on the history, the findings, and upon a consideration of the possibilities which may produce a similar picture. Family counseling must be preceded by a history of the problem and of the developmental processes which produced the family in its present state (1). If we misjudge the factors which lead to and maintain the disturbance, we may also fail to assess the potential for change and falter in selecting the area upon which we should focus our efforts. Family counseling is a form of marriage therapy, because the marital couple shapes the family as they evolve into parental roles. After clarifying the problem, the physician can take his history of the family by beginning at the natural point, when the mates first met each other. In a casual, yet attentive manner, he collects his data on the development of the relationship through courtship and into marriage, allowing a variety of emotions to be ventilated as they are stimulated by memories. In a sense, the therapeutic effects of the counseling begin with the history-taking phase. In a thorough manner, the physician should become aware of every member of the family, and the influence of peripheral, but important relatives influencing the family patterns. Therefore, the relationship of each mate to his own parents and to the in-laws must be included. When discrepancies exist between the points of view of the husband and wife on historical facts, the physician can begin to improve their communication by examining the cause of their misunderstanding. Helping them to see the different ways they have reacted to their own parents and the fact that their parents were different personalities, introduces the concept of different-ness (8). The physician can have each mate clarify the similarities and differences between them and the techniques they use to adapt to these qualities. The value of the history now becomes apparent, for the counselor may find a relationship between the methods used by the couple and the patterns they observed in their own parents. The patients may be reacting with an opposite pattern as a rejection of the parental behavior, but still inappropriate for each other, or they may be using a repetitious technique reflecting their own parent-child or sibling relationship. Thus, without introducing the psychoanalytic concept of transference, couples can begin to gain some insight into their interpersonal reactions. The physician helps each of the marital partners view similar material in their history in order to coordinate the subject matter of the same developmental period and thereby compare their individual experiences. In reviving memories of their original family life, the couple can empathize more readily with the experiences their children are now having in the present family situation. Families in trouble find it just as difficult to reveal their pleasurable experiences as to discuss their areas of conflict. Therefore, information should also be elicited in the areas of their family and marital pleasures.

The emphasis upon influences from the past diminishes the tendency of couples to fix blame upon each other and increases the chance for them to begin an understanding approach to the problem. Their expectations from marriage is another crucial area for exploration and counseling. The manner in which disappointments and hopes are communicated and the techniques each used to deal with his or her feelings are often an important source of disturbance in the family. Counseling must stimulate a gradual acceptance of the imperfections and differences among human beings. Each mate can learn from family counseling that he has had some meaningful responsibility in his selection of the other for marriage. They may have concealed or disguised their needs from themselves or each other and thus set the stage for the other partner's failure in the relationship.

Their feelings about having children, the events that occurred during each child's development, and the various feelings of each family member toward the other are explored. The general picture described in the foregoing permits the physician to become oriented to the family problem and encourages the family toward an objectivity modeled after the physician's approach. He can then decide which area needs his attention first, picking his clues from the family, and actively encouraging family explorations into the area of disturbance. After seeing the marital couple for a few sessions, children are introduced into the family counseling, although, as I expressed earlier, the family combinations vary with the situation. The control of young children in the session is usually best left with the parents. The physician helps the parents see and understand the child's feelings and helps the child accept the differences in his parents. Parents can learn a great deal about their own behavior patterns from seeing themselves through their child's eyes. Although the physician doing family counseling should support parental authority, he can help parents recognize the increasing maturity of their child for accepting certain appropriate responsibilities.

Thus far I have described a basic method for instituting family counseling. When the family is actively involved in the process of learning to look at themselves, rather than finding others to blame, the physician has certain techniques available to him. The physician's ability to get to the facts helps the family see a direction to the interviews and helps them to realize that they have something of value to contribute to the treatment. In effect, the therapist helps the family become aware of the importance of clear, direct communication. His inquiry into their daily lives includes an open discussion about their sex activities. The subject of sex must be dealt with in the same objective, non-judgmental manner as other aspects of life. People tend to say one thing, but confuse their communications by double-level messages in which their behavior is not consistent with their words. The physician who can recognize confused communication among family members makes this observation to each person as it occurs. Those who are more experienced in psychotherapeutic techniques know that patients will accept an honest, forthright opinion when it is constructive, appropriate and helpful. However, the counselor must also point out the assets of a patient and foster his confidence and self-esteem by his respect and value for the patient's opinions and feelings. In the family counseling method, the physician must be alert to and interfere with the tendency of certain family members to speak for another, thus encouraging individuality for each person, yet taking care not to assume a biased position toward anyone in the group. He must also remain watchful of those who remain silent, for, in a family setting, it implies hidden controls wherein the silent member feels it is dangerous to assert himself in the presence of someone in the family.

This issue leads to another important point, namely, families in trouble are often preoccupied with fears of being hurt or hurting each other. Thus, they are defensive in their relationship to protect their self-esteem. Anger is a common defense against feeling helpless, vulnerable, and hurt. A family counselor can help families look beneath the hostility and investigate the areas of their sensitivity, as well as diminish their fears of hurting others when they are self-assertive or communicating observations. In general the physician must help families see their multiple roles of responsibility to themselves as individuals, to their mate within a marriage, and as parents.

In the foregoing, I have touched upon various aspects of family counseling. Family researchers tend to focus on specific areas, such as the fixed patterns of interaction, the communication processes, or the discordance between overt behavior and inner feelings. In agreement with all theories, one can see that families must find means for adapting to the discrepancies that are inevitable within and between individuals (4). Disturbances in a family member usually serve some purpose for the family unit, in other words, it reflects an attempt to adapt to something happening in the family (9). The family equilibrium would be considered pathological under such circumstances. If the disturbed person is successfully treated without changing the family scheme, the patient will either create a new state of family dysfunction, will lapse back into his previous pathology, or someone else in the family will become disturbed. On the other hand, healthy families apparently utilize mechanisms which deal with relationship problems in ways that are not pathogenic for its members. Their conflicts seem to be self-limiting, occur upon a foundation of family solidarity and are kept within their own family boundaries, avoiding extension into peripheral relatives (3). It is known that the family in our country usually establishes itself on an independent basis with clearly defined boundaries (7). Disturbed families tend to have vague boundaries and more often involve parents and in-laws or other relatives in their conflicts and tensions. The relatives tend to take sides, to amplify and prolong the problem. The family counselor should be aware of this tendency in a disturbed family and avoid becoming entangled with the relatives, which may lead to a hopeless confusion in dealing with the problem. Thus, the therapist must maintain an optimal distance and relate *to* the family, and not act as if he were an extended part of the family. He can encourage the family to establish its boundaries if the relatives respond in a pathological manner.

Returning to my original statement, family counseling is really "old hat" to the physician who is a trusted friend to his patient. The intent of this presentation was to briefly convey the methodology that has been developed out of the cumulative experience of a number of psychotherapists who work within the framework of family psychodynamics. Physicians who may not be in a position to continue family counseling over a long series of consecutive meetings can offer meaningful help to their patients with this interviewing technique. The physician who sets the stage for the family to expose its patterns of interaction will experience a sense of gratification in viewing a vivid display of psychic mechanisms which gradually leads toward the diminution of each member's painful anxiety. As a consultation experience, it provides the physician a better means of determining whether a member of the family needs more specific individual psychiatric therapy. The person who is most pained in the family may not be the sick member.

In addition to serving as a *diagnostic* and *therapeutic* instrument, the family interview may be useful as a *teaching* method in clinics to demonstrate the forces which act upon a given patient. A psychiatric resident who observed a family interview that I conducted was asked to record his own reactions to this experience. He wrote, "In my limited experience it could only be matched in intimacy by the final twenty minutes of *Tea and Sympathy*. As a matter of fact, although the contents were loosely related, the session contrasted with the theater in at least two ways. First, there was no plot, in the usual sense, to carry one along to a dramatic climax; it was more akin to perceiving an entire painting almost immediately and then having the colors become steadily more vivid and hypnotic. Secondly, it was impossible to intermittantly relieve one's anxiety—to find momentary respite in the thought that this was dramatic theater and though realistic, not real. Nor could the reality be shrugged off as insanity, for while there were considerable amounts of pathology demonstrated, none of it could be called psychotic." The case which he witnessed involved an eighteen-year-old boy who had been individually treated by a series of psychiatrists for a severe obsessive-compulsive neurosis and learning problem.† His mother and father were both professional people. The father received treatment for a year in a psychiatric hospital four years ago. When they entered for their first family interview, the mother was followed by the patient, his twelve-year-old sister and the father. They selected their own seating arrangement, which was son, mother, daughter, and father. The mother and son were impeccably dressed in contrast to the father and daughter who appeared quite plain. The father frequently caressed his daughter's hand and they exchanged humorous glances at times suggesting a long standing semi-secret alliance. My brief opening remarks to the family expressed awareness of the pain they were experiencing and my interest in knowing how their family functions. They were told that having them all together offers us the opportunity to obtain a clearer picture of their family. The questions then were directed toward clarifying the problem as each saw it. Later the questions moved toward taking a history of the development of the family as described earlier in this paper. In this case, the father immediately deferred to his wife, but I encouraged him to speak for himself, that his thoughts as head of the family were important to each of us. In this manner I attempted to begin the process of helping him reestablish his family status, identity, and self-esteem. His response was forceful as he went into a long, highly intellectualized attempt to dissect the problem, revealing intense rage at his son and wife. The therapist's role here is to help each one clarify

---

† The author recently completed a pilot study of family interaction in a series of cases where the adolescent member had a learning problem (6).

their communications. The father tried to defend his status and protect his self-esteem by assuming the position of the greatest intellect and prided himself in the fact that few people could understand his complex, circumstantial thinking. The mother described her son's problem as having its origin in early childhood due to the competitiveness between herself and her mother for the patient's affection. The son quickly became involved in a running conflict with his father answering the father's attack upon him during the initial description of the problem. The mother began to serve as moderator between her husband and son, primarily comforting her son, and at one point she suddenly turned towards him and said, "Let's face it; I love you and I'm very jealous." This had been provoked by the father's accusations regarding her protective attitude toward her son. The father's reaction to her statement was one of stoic rigidity—he didn't bat an eyelash. I asked him if his expression meant he was surprised. Here the intention was to help them practice clear, one-level communication. He answered that he knew she loved him and maybe that was part of the trouble—he can't become a man because he is still her baby. The son immediately denied this as a cause of the problem and stated that his illness started when they began to move from city to city during his childhood. Thus, he turned the blame on the father's occupational problems. In the meanwhile, the mother was gently carressing her son's hand to comfort him, but her attention was actually increasing his anxiety. At a later point the father criticized his son for no longer being interested in world affairs. This represented one area of the father's interest and reflected his feeling of rejection by his son. The son pointed out that this lack of present interest was true, but he attributed this to his being behind in school and wanting to focus what little power of concentration he had available on his school sujects. This response made the father feel supportive for the first time and he told about the problem he experienced with a thesis he wrote. At another point the father remarked, "I don't think my son is a schizophrenic." This was in reference to a diagnosis once given by one of their earlier psychiatrists, but was nonetheless in contrast with the father's previous pattern of using this label to attack his son. At the end of this sixty-minute session, the father said to his son, "This is the first time in years you've talked to me like this." His son replied, "I never knew you felt this way."

The time and space limitations preclude any systematic exploration of the family dynamics in this brief vignette. One can see the focal symbiosis of a mother-son and father-daughter pairing, the oedipal problems and regressions in each member to defend against their incestuous feelings as well as the way each parent used a child to defend against their fears of relating to each other. In addition there were sado-masochistic patterns established in several directions. The family interview became a stimulus to deal with some of the ego-syntonic resistances that prevented individual therapy from making much progress. Using this method, the therapist can better define the role each family member is covertly playing with the others and whether it is appropriate for their family position. He can promote communication which allows members to say and act consistently with what they feel, and to discover the earlier models upon which their behavior is based.

Finally, I think it is warranted to point out to physicians who may have some experience or awareness of group psychotherapy that family counseling is not to be misconstrued as group therapy (2, 5). The family has its fixed patterns established before seeking help and the techniques and goals in therapy are directed toward promoting healthy integration of the group. In contrast, group therapy utilizes an artificially created group to promote their interaction for a limited period of time for the purpose of helping the individuals with their personal problems. In family counseling, the meetings are part of their continuing family life, and the effects of the therapy can be promoted by the group during the intervals between therapy sessions. Each family must be helped to find the healthiest pattern for its situation, enhance its own identity and strength, as well as provide the members with security as individuals.

REFERENCES

1. Ackerman, Nathan W.: *The Psychodynamics of Family Life.* New York, Basic Books, Inc., 1958, Chap. 9.

2. Bell, John E.: A theoretical position for family group therapy. *Family Process, 2*:1-14, 1963.
3. Bell, Norman W.: Extended family relations of disturbed and well families. *Family Process, 1*:175-193, 1962.
4. Jackson, D. D.: Family interaction, family homeostasis, and some implications for conjoint family psychotherapy. In J. Masserman (Ed.), *Individual and Familial Dynamics*. New York, Grune & Stratton, 1959.
5. Marcus, Irwin M.: Psychoanalytic Group Therapy with Fathers of Emotionally Disturbed Preschool Children. *Int. J. Group Psychother., 6*:61-76, 1956.
6. ——————: Family interaction in Adolescents with learning difficulties. Phase I of a pilot study. Presented at the 1965 Annual Meeting of the *American Orthopsychiatric Association.*
7. Parsons, Talcott: The kinship system of the contemporary United States. In Parsons, Talcott: *Essay in Sociological Theory*. Glencoe Free Press, 1954.
8. Satir, Virginia: *Conjoint Family Therapy*. Calif., Science and Behavior Books, Inc., 1964.
9. Vogel, Ezra F., and Bell, Norman W.: The emotionally disturbed child as a family scapegoat. *Psychoanalysis, 47*:21-42, 1960.

PSYCHIATRY AND THE SURGEON

M. L. MICHEL, M.D.

Discussions of psychiatric problems associated with surgical care have previously focused on intrinsic disorders in the patient. The emotional impact of major operations on both stable and unstable patients has been well documented, and psychiatric complications before and after operations have been adequately described, particularly in psychiatric publications. Little attention has been given, however, to emotional instability and psychiatric problems in surgeons themselves and the adverse emotional responses these can elicit in surgical patients. Similarly, emotional disturbances of anesthesiologists, consultants, resident physicians, interns, medical students, nurses, and others who attend surgical patients may have deleterious effects on patients. Thus, adequate discussion of the subject should include (1) intrinsic psychiatric problems of surgical patients; (2) extrinsic factors, including (a) emotional problems of surgeons and (b) emotional problems of ancillary surgical personnel.

INTRINSIC PSYCHIATRIC PROBLEMS OF SURGICAL PATIENTS

The surgeon should consider the potential psychiatric problems of his patients from the first visit to their discharge. An operation produces stress in even an emotionally stable patient and can create a serious disturbance in the patient who already has a psychiatric disorder. The surgeon's failure to recognize these possibilities can cause complications and even death.

Psychiatric problems associated with elective operations can be more severe and prolonged than those associated with

141

emergency operations. The preoperative period for an elective operation allows the patient time to ponder possible untoward effects and thus creates anxiety and stress. By emphasizing the lack of urgency for the operation and by taking advantage of the longer preoperative period to prepare the patient psychologically, the surgeon can usually achieve the patient's intellectual acceptance of the operation. In emergency operations, on the other hand, little time is available for preoperative psychologic preparation by the surgeon or adjustment by the patient; the magnitude or severity of physical signs and symptoms may obliterate the surgeon's consideration of emotional factors. The surgeon should discuss the operation and its effects adequately to satisfy the curiosity of adult patients and of parents of pediatric patients. He should, however, guard against going into excessive detail with the patient who already has an anxiety neurosis.

For individual evaluation of each patient, the surgeon may divide his patients into three major classes: (1) stable; (2) neurotic or potentially psychotic, and (3) psychotic. Since most surgeons have limited knowledge of psychiatry, they may have difficulty making such a simplified classification. Several informal interviews with the patient before the operation, during which he is allowed to talk freely of his anxieties, may help the surgeon uncover any signs of instability or other special problems. Pointed questioning about the patient's psychiatric status, on the other hand, may create resentment, aggravate any existing psychiatric problem, and jeopardize the surgeon-patient relation.

Interestingly, most neurotic patients behave well during operative experiences. Possibly the real problems associated with an operation furnish an effective substitute for the numerous imaginary problems of their everyday lives. Neurotic surgical patients, however, require more reassurance and understanding from the surgeon than stable patients. The surgeon must realize that many neurotic, and even some psychotic patients enjoy being operated on. Even when their physical condition is not improved by the operation, the mental effects are often salutary, at least temporarily.

For this reason, the surgeon should be particularly cautious about patients with multiple abdominal incisions and should review the patient's previous hospital records carefully to determine if the operations were justified. The possible placebo effects of major operations have been well documented. The patient's subjective benefit far exceeds any objective improvement, but is usually only transient, disappearing after the surgeon discharges the patient. Such placebo effects are usually attributable to one of two sources: (1) emotional instability in the patient or (2) overenthusiasm by the surgeon.

Surgeons, as well as other trained specialists, can help eliminate such unnecessary operations. Certain operations on patients with minimal symptoms or pathologic change which may produce placebo effects and are difficult to evaluate include: hysterectomy, elective operations for abdominal adhesions, anorectal operations, removal of carotid sinus for asthma, operation for peptic ulcer, cholecystectomy, particularly in middle-aged women, and elective appendectomy for "chronic appendicitis."

When the surgeon cannot distinguish between psychosis and neurosis in a patient, he should seek the advice of a psychiatrist. If the patient is considered to be potentially psychotic, psychiatric consultation should be requested before operation and, if necessary, during the postoperative period. A latent psychosis may sometimes become aggravated before operation or, more often, after operation. The known psychotic patient should not be subjected to major surgical operation unless it is a life-saving procedure or unless symptoms and signs interfere with the patient's emotional adjustment. Many psychotic patients now become well stabilized after use of drugs and other psychiatric treatment. The usual indications for operations apply in these patients if the psychiatrist agrees that the psychiatric state will not be aggravated. The surgeon must guard against transference reaction by the patient who is receiving psychotherapy; such a response can interfere with psychotherapy and often veils the patient's genuine hostility toward the surgeon.

Emergency operations present a special problem. Time does not permit preoperative psychiatric evaluation. Prophylactic drugs and other measures should be used to protect the patient from the psychologic trauma of emergency diagnostic procedures. Ancillary personnel should be trained to avoid agitating the patient in any way. The surgeon should always appear calm, since any demonstration of concern about the patient's physical condition is easily communicated. As soon as possible after the operation, the surgeon should explain the nature of the illness and the operation, particularly if the patient is unstable. Evasion and deception should be avoided. These patients need more attention in the postoperative period than those who have had elective operations.

Even when a psychiatric patient is incoherent, the surgeon must realize that he can understand a great deal and must therefore be careful what he says in the patient's presence. Moreover, such a patient can often give valuable information about his surgical disease by answering specific, direct questions. Physical examination of emotionally disturbed patients should be conducted with particular care, since many of them are inordinately modest. The surgeon should also be aware of other abnormal reactions of these patients. Among these is defense-through-denial, which may occur in the period either before or after operation. Such a reaction is often seen in intelligent, educated women with far-advanced cancer of the breast. Adverse conditioning, as a result of a previous disturbing surgical experience, can often be corrected by patient explanation and understanding. Depression is another common psychiatric complication in unstable surgical patients, particularly during the postoperative period. Even an acute postoperative psychosis, with delirium and other symptoms, will usually clear with good nursing care and proper use of drugs and supportive therapy. If the patient is not already under psychiatric treatment, psychiatric consultation should be sought.

EMOTIONAL PROBLEMS OF SURGEONS

Most physicians today have made the proper choice of a speciality, but some find themselves trapped in a professional life for which they are not suited. In view of the shortage of physicians, every effort should be made to obtain maximum efficiency from available professional medical personnel. Medical educators are becoming more cognizant of this problem and are giving greater attention to guiding medical students and interns into specialities for which they have particular aptitude.

A program of psychologic evaluation and screening of medical students during their undergraduate medical career merits consideration. The department of psychiatry should direct such a program and should have the full cooperation of the other clinical departments. Whereas the academic potential of a student is fairly well known on his graduation, little is known about his emotional status. Stable students would welcome such counseling to enhance their future success and happiness. Those who object because they have major real or imaginary problems might well profit from early psychotherapy.

Medical students should be made more aware of psychosomatic aspects of various illnesses by devoting a larger proportion of the curriculum to instruction in psychiatry and by better integration of such instruction with teaching in other clinical subjects. Combined surgical-psychiatric conferences, for example, are rare today.

Surgery can be a stressful occupation. Surgical resident physicians should be selected on the basis not only of academic achievement and technical skill but also of emotional stability. In a Symposium on Residency Training at the annual meeting of the American College of Surgeons in 1964, it was suggested that prospective resident physicians be screened by formal psychologic testing. At present, psychiatry is the only speciality in which candidates for residency training are screened psychologically. We rely solely on informal and inexpert opinions regarding an applicant's suitability for a surgical career.

The problem of misfits already in surgical practice is, of course, more complex. If the emotional disturbances become serious enough, they may necessitate action by those in authority. Referring physicians should bear in mind that surgeons with serious emotional problems are unsuited to treat patients with psychiatric disorders. Closer integration between the departments of psychiatry and surgery in hospital activities might effect a better understanding of the emotional state of surgical patients and might make surgeons more aware of their own emotional problems. Young members of the hospital staff, especially, might then be more likely to seek or accept psychiatric aid when they need it.

EMOTIONAL PROBLEMS OF ANCILLARY SURGICAL PERSONNEL

The emotional status of a surgical patient can be affected not only by that of the surgeon but by that of ancillary attendants as well. Anesthesiologists, nurses, resident physicians, interns, and medical students are particularly influential, but radiologists, laboratory technicians, and even aides exert some effect.

The surgeon is obligated to protect the patient as much as possible from emotional trauma induced by any of the personnel attending him. Since many patients fear anesthesia more than the operation, a visit by the anesthesiologist on the evening preceding operation may help relieve the patient and his family of undue anxiety. Nurses in the operating room should be particularly careful of conversations that can be overheard by patients, and nurses in the recovery room should be similarly cautious. Because of the influence of certain drugs and anesthetic agents and because of the understandable state of anxiety, patients may misinterpret what they hear. The surgeon should continually emphasize to the house staff the importance of the psychologic aspects of an operation, in addition to the scientific and technical aspects. Particularly when the patient is known to have an emotional problem, the surgeon should explain the nature of the problem to all ancillary personnel and should advise them how to avoid aggravating the disturbance by additional psychic trauma.

SUMMARY

Psychiatric problems in the practice of surgery are numerous and complex. Intrinsic psychiatric problems of the patient have been well documented, but little attention has been given to two important extrinsic factors: the effect of emotional instability of the surgeon on the patient and possible emotional trauma to the patient by ancillary personnel.

The following suggestions are offered as means of improving the management of surgical patients with psychiatric problems: psychologic counseling of medical students to direct them into specialties for which they are emotionally suited, psychologic screening of applicants for surgical residencies, increase in time devoted to psychiatry in the undergraduate curriculum, closer integration of psychiatry with other clinical disciplines in both medical schools and hospitals, and special instruction to ancillary surgical personnel in handling psychiatric problems of surgical patients.

PANEL DISCUSSION

MODERATOR: THOMAS G. WEBSTER

PANELISTS: MICHEL, LAMBERT AND MARCUS

Dr. Webster:

To open the panel discussion, I wonder if we might hear directly from those of you in the audience who have questions or comments.

Audience:

Dr. Michel's presentation has certainly been scholarly. One point might be emphasized, and that has to do with fear and panic. I've had two recent patients who have had surgery and one of them had angina. He was middle aged and he developed severe bouts of abdominal pain that were due to gall stones. This was presented to him. He was an ideal surgical patient, and he was worked up thoroughly. I did not make rounds that night. About 9:00 p.m. he panicked and at 4:00 a.m. he developed a very massive anterior myocardial infarction and has not had the surgery to this day. He has gotten along very well. The second patient panicked on the way to the operating room. She was operated in a hospital to which I very seldom go and she didn't tell the surgeon or anyone about it. She developed tachycardia that was a postoperative complication.

Dr. Michel:

Fear of an operation was one important subject I did not have time to discuss. There has been much written about this

148

in the psychiatric literature, but very little in the surgical literature.

There are three types of fear that a patient may have before undergoing an operation: (1) fear of mutilation (frequent in women prior to breast operations); (2) fear of pain, and (3) fear of death, which is the most common type.

In discussions with the patient before operation, by allowing the patient to "ventilate," the surgeon can frequently detect abnormal fear. If this is excessive, psychiatric help is necessary. If the fear is slight, an internist or generalist, who is familiar with the patient, can usually handle the situation.

Patients with excessive fear should be heavily sedated. I also use tranquilizing drugs, particularly Vistaril®. This is the safest drug of this type in the immediate pre- and postanesthetic period.

Audience:

In order for a surgical patient to give a well-informed consent and in order to forestall malpractice claims, you're supposed to outline all the ghastly and gory complications possible. What effect do you think this has on his psyche?

Dr. Michel:

It is inadvisable to discuss beforehand the possible complications that a patient may have following an operation. I do not discuss these unless the patient specifically asks for such information. It is important, however, in debatable operative procedures where the results are uncertain, not to mislead the patient.

Dr. Marcus:

I also would like to point out the problem of surgeons going into too great detail with patients telling them how much blood is involved, about soaking up clots and other gory aspects of surgery.

Dr. Michel:

I agree that discussion of the details of an operation should never take place on the night before surgery. Such gory details as listed by Dr. Marcus should not be described even to physician patients.

Audience:

I had a hemorrhoidectomy last summer. I was telling an internist about it right afterwards. He said, "Surgeons just don't psychologically prepare their patients." I agreed with him, because of the pain.

Dr. Michel:

The psychosomatic elements of anorectal surgery are important. This is something that deserves more attention from surgeons.

Relief of pain is also important in these cases. The patient should not be misled before operation as to the degree of post-operative pain which is to be expected.

Dr. Lambert:

I'd like to make a little more specific something that has been implicit throughout these two days. The medical practitioner plays an important role in preventive work, by anticipatory guidance, and preparation of the patient for oncoming events or procedures. Many times it's nice to know that the door is going to slam before it does slam. You're a little less startled. Certainly in working with children and working with adolescents a little preparation for what is coming can be most reassuring, not only to the child, the adolescent, but to the parent. And I think similarly in terms of surgical procedures some anticipatory guidance diminishes the amount of distress at the time.

Just as preoperative support and reassurance is indicated so is post-operative support and reassurance important. It has been noted that where patients are seen in the recovery room following general anesthesia, during the first twenty-four hours they show very little emotional concern. The following day however, they show considerable irritability and anxiety which can be allayed by visits from the family physician or surgeon if there has been a good preoperative relationship.

Dr. Webster:

I think there have been two points made here that merit some elaboration. On the one hand there is a place for anticipatory guidance and for preparing a patient for surgery. On the other hand, it can be overdone. I wonder if we can hear some discussion about the guidelines a physician might follow. What factors might you assess in the patient in order to guide you as to when you are unnecessarily scaring the patient with details as compared to when the patient needs a little more information. Maybe some of you from your practice experience could comment.

Audience:

I say this from my personal experience, if they had gone into too much I might not have had the hemorrhoidectomy.

Audience:

I think a good deal of this depends upon knowing the patient. When I've known a patient twenty-five years and he develops a surgical condition, I'm going to guide him. Recently we had a patient who had been in psychotherapy for quite some time. She developed pain and this pain turned out to be due to a stone in a common duct. By knowing the patient and knowing the fact that she was hysterical and manic, the surgeon and I were able to guide her through her surgery without any difficulty. She was a very fine patient.

Dr. Marcus:

This reminded me of a situation. Some years ago I had a woman who was under psychoanalytic treatment. As you know, in analytic treatment you go into detail about the person's fantasy life and memories. She was an unmarried woman, in her forties, and expressed regrets that she hadn't married and her longing for children. During this period she came in and said, "I have a terrible pain in my stomach. I've been disturbed with it all night." She proceeded to try to convince me that this was due to her desire for a baby. I asked her about the disturbance during the night and what her feelings were in the morning and whether or not she had breakfast. I didn't examine her, but in asking her about her pain, she described it in the epigastrium. She expected me to accept her theory that this was part of her pregnancy wish. There is always the possibility that a psychiatric patient can develop physical disturbances such as appendicitis. I called her physician and made arrangements for him to see her. She was operated that day. She had an acute appendicitis.

Dr. Michel:

Concerning preoperative discussions with surgical patients, the internist or the general practitioner may have adequately discussed what is going to be done at operation. In such a situation the surgeon's discussion with the patient can be curtailed.

However, the surgeon should still visit the patient and at least chat with him before operation, even though the details of the operative procedure may have been explained by another consultant.

Dr. Lambert:

The surgeon in talking with the patient might be guided in how much to explain to the patient by satisfying the patient's curiosity and at the same time avoid stimulating the curiosity. For instance, he will say to the patient, "Do you have any questions?" Then he gives a brief simple answer. If it is satisfying, fine. If the patient is not satisfied he will ask further questions. The patient, in other words, gives you a guideline as to how far to go.

Audience:

To either Dr. Lambert or Dr. Marcus. In my neighborhood a good many adolescents have the habit of coming into the office. I think they talk about it among themselves. They tell the receptionist they are coming in because of a "cold." When they enter my office they immediately say, "Now this is the problem that I want to talk to you about. I'm going to pay for it out of my allowance. Don't talk to my parents." Just what is my spot there? Sometimes one doesn't have to talk to their parents. Sometimes, one should.

Dr. Marcus:

What was the age group you were referring to?

Audience:

Primarily fifteen to eighteen.

Dr. Marcus:

I feel that the physician has a responsibility to the family. I think the physician should point out that discussions are medical treatment. Psychotherapy is medical treatment. Therefore, you're risking medical treatment upon a minor without parental permission. Although the people in the nonmedical field get around this by saying, well we're not really doing treatment. We're only doing guidance work or counseling, and so forth. I feel that the adolescent should be oriented to the fact that in order to have medical treatment, the parent must give permission. I would assure them that this does not mean that the parent would necessarily be told any secrets unless it involved a serious threat to their mental or physical well-being. I don't think it's a good idea to enter into alliances that would place you out on a limb when you really need the family's help in the situation. The situation may stem from the child's irrational, neurotic fear which may be inappropriate in terms of family situation. The child's request is part of the rift that might be taking place at the time and perhaps part of the rebellion and hatred they might be experiencing. I think the physician can help the situation if he enters into it on a sound basis.

Dr. Lambert:

This is the point I've tried to make. Not to get caught between the parent and the child. I think you can help the child by indicating that since they are legally a minor (you may not put it in those terms), that they are dependent on the parent. It has to be recognized though they may be trying to emancipate themselves by setting up their own individual appointment. You can encourage the adolescent to tell his family about wanting to see you and that you'll be glad to discuss anything off the record, but it should be with the understanding that the family must know of the visit.

Audience:

Just two interesting points. One is psychiatrists have all had the experience of treating one mate, with her making sure, or having us ascertain that we will not tell the other mate. I think this is quite cricket. Although certainly a goal in therapy should be to get the mate to communicate to the other mate that she is undergoing therapy, I think you do honor her wish and try to help this person with her problem. Another thing concerns college students. Many university health services offer psychiatric psychotherapy with the assurance to the college student that if the college student does not want the communication to the parent, they will not communicate unless the patient becomes significantly disturbed (of course, that word "significantly disturbed" can be interpreted many ways) or requires psychiatric hospitalization. I do think that many of the health services do go along with maintaining the confidence of the child. Again, the goal should be to have the communication system set up whereby they can communicate with those who are responsible for them. Maybe Dr. Lambert would know how it is done in the East. I think Harvard does it this way without their being of legal age, and I'm quite sure Tulane does it this way.

Dr. Lambert:

As far as I know there has never been any issue about the age of a student when he consults (a psychiatrist or the Mental Health Services) within the student health services of a college or university. This may be because relatively few are below the age of eighteen and when they are it is possible the school is seen in *loco parentis*. Furthermore, the student is always assured of confidentiality. The psychiatrist never divulges any information except with the express permission of the student and even then would take up matters in general terms with the administration or parents so as to permit collaborative efforts to resolve the problem.

Dr. Michel:

I'd like to ask for discussion by the psychiatrists concerning psychological screening of applicants for surgical residencies.

Screening of residency applicants is done in psychiatry. Is it possible for us to do the same in surgery?

Dr. Marcus:

I think that a move toward having psychiatric evaluation for residents in all fields should be undertaken with considerable caution, and I'll tell you why I feel this way. It's very easy to become over-enthusiastic about psychiatric evaluation, and I think that the more a person has had experiences of seeing people helped by psychiatry, the more it encourages the enthusiasm. On the other hand, we have to consider, as we would in any branch of medicine, certain scientific principles. One of these principles is the fact that you don't have any standards. You don't have any norms. You don't know what kind of a personality is healthy for a surgeon, an eye specialist or an obstetrician. I would certainly be opposed to anyone pretending to know things that we don't really know. The fact is there probably are any number of oustanding surgeons—I'm going to pick surgery because you've introduced it as surgery—some of whom I know from experiences here and elsewhere whose personalities might not have been acceptable. Their patients will tell you that Dr. so and so doesn't have any bedside manner. But they would want to be operated by him any time they need it. There are any number of physicians who feel this way about the surgeons they have confidence in. They know that the individual may be a person whose personality might not be as flexible or less warm than they'd like, nevertheless, the men are very capable and have made important contributions. The first issue that would occur to me is, what is the range of personality types—whether it be for surgery or for any aspect of medical practice—that is considered healthy or acceptable.

I would agree that if any screening were to be considered,

perhaps the first stage would merely screen out the people that are psychotic. I don't think we want to get psychotic people involved in certain fields, or probably any of the fields.

Now I'd like to tell you about one situation, because it's very unusual. It had to do with a surgeon who was female and who had, over a period of time, successfully amputated both of her own breasts. During this period of time she was carrying on an active surgical practice. She was in a psychotic state (this is where psychosis is dangerous for a physican)—she had fantasies which were parallel with her own medical knowledge. You can have unconscious irrational thoughts existing side by side with what you've acquired intellectually as valid knowledge. Her fantasied wish was to convert herself into a male, and this was the reason she went through these procedures.

Audience:

In a lighter vein, I agree with Dr. Marcus. Dr. Michel may wish to read a serious article that appeared several years ago which analyzed the personalities of various types of medical specialists. I recall that they described the surgeon, by and large, as being people who are basically and subconsciously sadistic and that subconsciously they have the desire to inflict pain and then to heal people up. So actually it might not be such a good idea to dig too deeply into the psychological mechanisms of prospective surgeons.

Dr. Michel:

I agree that any type of screening has limitations. However, as far as possible, we would like to prevent psychotics and severe neurotics from entering surgical residencies.

If an applicant is stable, he can usually make his own choice of a specialty without counselling. However, we would like to make some effort to prevent emotionally disturbed people from getting into surgery. These individuals give us more trouble than all of our other problems combined, whether they be residents or practitioners.

Dr. Marcus:

Incidentally, in psychiatry we have as many, or more severely disturbed people as in any specialty I know. I'm not saying this critically. I'm telling you this because I've been involved in the training of psychiatrists since 1949 and I can tell you that there are a considerable percentage that make good psychiatrists. But there are any number of them that do get through the screenings. There are many reasons for it. It depends upon what center is doing the training. The centers that get less applicants for residency are less particular. Even though they think of themselves as being particular. If they have three applicants and all three are seriously neurotic, somehow or other they rationalize their acceptance. We try to eliminate the psychotics, but I know of any number of psychiatrists who went through training, who were psychotic when they went in and were psychotic when they came out.

It depends upon what happens with their psychosis, whether they are completely out in left field or whether they manage in some way to keep reasonable controls on themselves with regard to behavior with patients. I just wanted you to know that psychiatry is not immune to having very seriously disturbed members.

Dr. Webster:

Well, I'm relieved to know that if we're going to get into the personality problems of physicians, that we have centered on the professions represented on the panel rather than on those of the audience! I think a number of very interesting points have been raised which are relevant to professional training. I think that with the little time we have remaining, we might focus on questions relating to patients in general medical practice.

Audience:

If the specialties get psychotic physicians screened out, are you going to leave them for general practice?

Dr. Webster:

I thought I was going to head this discussion off before that implication came up!

Dr. Lambert:

I think it probably takes a more solid, stable, emotionally

well-adjusted person to be a good general practitioner than probably any specialty that we have and certainly as much as many of the more complicated specialties.

Dr. Marcus:

Some of the warmest people that I've met in the field of medicine were in general practice. They are frequently the most relaxed with their patients, most considerate, and the original family psychiatrist.

Dr. Webster:

This afternoon Dr. Marcus talked about dealing with families. I would be interested to hear some of the experiences that many of you have had as to just how this works out in practice. I am sure that you have problems come up with a given patient in which the family is very much involved. What are some of the kinds of problems you encounter?

Audience:

I'd like to ask Dr. Lambert, particularly, to comment on the rising incidence of venereal disease among teenagers of this country. Are we having a moral breakdown, or just what is the score?

Dr. Lambert:

I don't know what the incidence is, whether there's just more awareness of the problem, whether it's just more in the open than it was in the past, whether it's an absolute increase or only a relative increase—I frankly don't know. I am reminded, however, of a story in line with what Dr. Usdin spoke of today in terms of the child telling what father does. The Commissioner of Health was a dermatologist and was responsible for venereal disease control in New York State. One day his six-year old daughter said, "Daddy's responsible for all the syphillis in the state." There is no question that we are in a period of marked change socially, culturally, economically, politically, and that values and standards are shifting. I know of no objective data on which to base the opinion about "moral breakdown." Impressionistically, many believe that there is more open sexual experimentation and activity. Undoubtedly, the development of medication to prevent pregnancy is a factor. It is perhaps more open than it used to be. I would suspect that if one thinks back to their own adolescent period and recalls what was going on in the peer group then, such activity was much less open but I frankly don't know if there was less then than now.

Audience:

I'd be interested in what Dr. Marcus thinks about that, too—in the change of sexual standards for the adolescents.

Dr. Marcus:

I feel that there is continuing change. There were early studies of sexual patterns in college women conducted in the 1920's. The percentage of college seniors who engage in sexual experience has gradually increased since then. I have not personally conducted statistical surveys. The bulk of my time is confined to private practice and as consultant to certain agencies in town. It looks as if there's a gradual increase in the curve with regard to the percentage of college females that are engaging in complete sexual experience. I don't think it's an alarming figure. It seems to be a reflection of the total change in our culture. The novels are using bold language and descriptions of various types of sexuality which are widely read, nationally and internationally; television programs are very mildly disguising some of the same type of material. The oral contraceptives may have contributed to the increased freedom.

One change that I've noticed over the past fifteen years is that the college boys were less likely to select the college girls and more likely to select other girls in the community for sexual activity, frequently those that were professional. Kinsey stated that the college girls that engaged in sexual experience were more likely to be engaged in sex that didn't involve the men on the campus. Their experiences involved men elsewhere or a certain percentage were with married men. Now there seems to be more involvement of the college boys with the college girls. They seem less afraid of their reputation. I don't know if this would hold as a valid observation on a national scale.

Audience:

Is that psychiatrically good or bad?

Dr. Marcus:

I think your question was a very good question. I don't know the answer, and I don't know what this really means. If people engaged in sexuality which might be potentially dangerous to them either socially or physically, it becomes a problem. Many girls who are engaged in premature sexual experiences feel very insecure and are not doing this because they're so "sexy," but because they're so insecure and want to feel something in the way of closeness as a substitute for love.

On the other hand, there are probably a small percentage that are not engaged in sexual activity out of insecurity but perhaps as a reflection of maturation and development. I think we will have to evaluate sex behavior on an individual basis and cannot generalize about it.

You know that sexual attitudes are different in foreign countries. I think that the "goodness or badness" has to be evaluated on a relative basis, relative to our culture, because what might be good for another culture could be bad in our culture. If the culture states, "go ahead and have sex," then, of course, people having premarital sex do not receive social rejection. I don't think our culture has reached that point.

Audience:

By either sex?

Dr. Marcus:

Our culture has a double standard. Our culture has, for years, encouraged men to have sex before marriage. It goes back into our history. All you have to do is walk though the French

Quarter and look at the construction of the buildings and you will see the bachelor quarters that were attached to old homes. These quarters were designed to permit late teenage sons to bring their girl friends up the back stairway and not disturb the family. In other words, men have always been encouraged to have premarital sexual experience. How they have this experience and what this experience means to them will be determined by family attitudes which involve many things, such as, social, economic, religious, and educational values.

Audience:

Along those lines, I have seen a number of pregnant high school teenagers from families that I have known. Some of them have an abortion. Some of them I have delivered. The parents want to know what to do. Should she stay home and have the baby? Should she go off? Should she get married? What's your opinion on this? What would you advise? Should she go off and have the baby somewhere else, like the Volunteers of America or the Catholic Home? Should she stay home—sometimes they want to stay home but the parents don't want them to stay there. Should she place the child for adoption? A lot of problems arise out of this, and they ask the family physician. I usually refer them to the clergyman, but I just want to know your opinion.

Dr. Marcus:

First of all, I would evaluate the total situation because usually a marriage for a fifteen-year-old girl is not going to solve her problem. Usually, it's going to compound the situation. Ordinarily, I wouldn't be advising that unless there were clear indications for an exception. Adolescents at fifteen are emotionally quite unstable and immature. They're not ready to take care of babies. They're certainly not ready to maintain a household, although there may be exceptions. So in having the baby the question is whether she should have it locally or go elsewhere. This involves a social issue in terms of how the family feels and whether or not such information will be common knowledge.

As far as abortions are concerned, I would never advise an abortion.

Audience:

Because of the impact on the girl?

Dr. Marcus:

I think that it does have far-reaching effects. I have treated women who told me about premarital abortions. In fact, I've had more than one woman tell me this in the course of treatment. And it does have an intense disturbing effect upon a woman to have her baby destroyed. I think that if she has her baby and it's handled in a healthy way, whereby she receives emotional support, she can accept adoption as a better approach for herself and the baby.

Dr. Webster:

I'd like to add one final comment regarding some of the kinds of questions that have come up. Very often, I think, psychiatric teachers and consultants are at their best when discussing individual cases.

We are grateful to our panel this afternoon for tackling some very tough general issues which are of concern to all practicing physicians. Psychiatrists obviously do not have all the answers to such complex matters, but they can sometimes be quite helpful in identifying the crucial facts in a given case and offering a way to deal with complex social and emotional factors more effectively. I hope that the nonspychiatric physicians present will have future opportunities for more individualized training and more intimate collaboration with psychiatrists on their own specific patients.

To the panel and to the audience, thank you very much for your participation.

PSYCHOPHARMACOLOGIC THERAPY FOR THE MEDICAL PRACTITIONER: CLINICAL ADVANTAGES AND DISADVANTAGES*

D. M. GALLANT, M.D.

IN CLINICAL DRUG research, the difficult and complex question that should be asked is, "Is the drug more efficacious than placebo?" This question still brings forth many confused answers. Therefore, before considering specific drugs available in psychopharmacologic therapy, it is necessary first to review briefly the value of placebo in research and clinical practice.

PLACEBO IN RESEARCH AND THERAPEUTICS

In the recent medical literature, definitions of placebo have been expanded. Based on historic criteria, a placebo is here defined as any therapeutic technic or inert pharmacologic preparation which is employed to have an effect on a symptom or disease without specific pharmacologic or therapeutic activity for the condition being treated. The placebo is also used as a control measure in research. In double-blind trials, the use of placebo as the most dependable method of testing the efficacy of drugs is well recognized. It must also be realized that double-blind trials are limited; it is almost impossible to fulfill the requirement that a placebo must conform to the medicine tested in every way *excluding* the therapeutic effect it produces. The

* Supported by Public Health Service Grant MH-5-T1-03701-06-A1 (Psychopharmacology Service Center, NIMH).

ideal tests include the comparisons of placebo to the standard (prototype) and trial preparations as well as the comparison of both preparations with one another.

The alteration of neurologic and psychic pain in many well controlled evaluations of placebo response leave no doubt as to the importance of the placebo reaction. Placebo responses in various headache studies have ranged from approximately 60 per cent in tension headache studies to 33 per cent in migraine studies. The outstanding postoperative analgesic experiments of Lasagna and his associates, which were conducted in 1954, have contributed greatly to placebo research (1). In an evaluation of 162 patients with postoperative pain, 31 per cent were consistent nonreactors to placebo, 14 per cent were consistent reactors, and 55 per cent reacted variably to placebos. It has been stated that the incidence of placebo reactions does not appear to be related to whether the patients are psychotic or neurotic although the intensity and range of such reactions may be greater in psychotics. However, in the studies conducted on the Tulane drug research ward and at Charity Hospital in New Orleans, a definite decrease in placebo effect has been found as the investigations changed from a neurotic population to a psychotic population. In the neurotic anxiety reactions, the placebo response ranges from 40 per cent to 60 per cent; in the neurotic depressive reactions, the placebo response occurs in 50 per cent to 80 per cent; in the acute schizophrenic studies, the placebo response is noted in 25 per cent to 50 per cent; and in the chronic schizophrenic studies, the placebo (or active placebo including phenobarbital) response ranges from 0 per cent to 10 per cent.

The placebo effect can actually reverse the normal pharmacologic action of a drug (2). For example, Wolf reports that his patient, Tom, was repeatedly given Prostigmin®, which induced abdominal cramps, diarrhea, hyperemia, hypersecretion and hypermotility of the stomach. Subsequently, the same response occurred not only to tap water and lactose capsules, but also to atropine sulfate which usually has an inhibiting effect on gastric function. It should be noted that Craighorn and his associates found that placebo had even greater effects on adrenal cortex functions of psychoneurotic patients as their anxiety increased (1). The changes which they observed were very similar to the changes produced in normal persons when they were administered ACTH; an increase of neutrophils, decrease in lymphocytes and eosinophils, and an increase of urinary keto-steroids. It is then apparent that even clinical biochemical investigations necessitate the use of a placebo group. These studies demonstrate the powerful effect of placebo. It can significantly modify the patient's functioning even to the extent of reversing the normal pharmacologic actions of drugs.

The following side effects associated with placebo therapy have been reported: sudden overwhelming weakness, palpitation, and nausea (3). Diffuse itchy erythema with maculopapular rashes are common, as well as epigastric pain, watery diarrhea, urticaria, edema of the lips, and dizziness. Severe headaches and multiple gastrointestinal complaints are frequent as a result of placebo administration. Drowsiness is the most common complaint. Thus, the relief of any particular symptom or exacerbation of any symptom by medication is not sufficient evidence of the specific effect of the drug unless it can be shown that this effect was not obtained as a placebo effect.

ANTIPSYCHOTIC COMPOUNDS

Phenothiazines

The main complications are granulocytopenia, dermatitis, abnormalities in liver function, and possibly seizures; the main side effects are extrapyramidal phenomena, visual disturbances, sedation, and orthostatic hypotension. No cases of true physiological addiction have been reported. The anti-cholinergic atropine-like activity may be uncomfortable for the patient but usually does not result in serious consequences (4).

In an extensive nine-hospital study of acute schizophrenics conducted by NIMH, the three major phenothiazine drugs investigated were Thorazine®, Prolixin®, and Mellaril® (6). In a double-blind study of 344 patients, these drugs were evaluated and compared to a placebo group. The overall therapeutic improvement for each of the three drug groups was approximately the same; 90 per cent of the patients showed mild to marked improvement at the end of six weeks. On the other hand, in the placebo group only 50 per cent showed mild to marked improvement at the end of six weeks. Other well controlled studies have shown similar results.

In the studies conducted on the Tulane research ward and at other drug investigation centers, it appears that Thorazine begins to reach therapeutic efficacy in gross psychotic schizophrenics at dosages of 200 mg daily, and no greater therapeutic efficacy is noted after the dosage reaches 1,000 mg daily. Stelazine reaches therapeutic efficacy in the same patient group at dosages of 6 to 8 mg daily, and no further improvement is noted after the maximum dosage has reached 30 mg daily.

Nonphenothiazines

An exciting new series of antipsychotic agents, the butyrophenone compounds (trifluperidol, haloperidol), is currently under investigation in several drug testing centers. During the past five years of double-blind studies on the Tulane Drug Research Ward, trifluperidol (daily dosage of 2 to 8 mg daily) was the only experimental drug to surpass Thorazine significantly in therapeutic efficacy (8, 9). Another impressive result was the relative lack of hypotensive and sedative side effects. The moderate extrapyramidal side effects can be adequately controlled with Cogentin 2 mg b.i.d. or t.i.d. However, these drugs have not yet been approved by the Federal Drug Administration.

ANTIDEPRESSANT COMPOUNDS

The main difficulty in perfoming an objective drug evaluation for therapeutic efficacy is best demonstrated with the antianxiety and antidepressant drug investigations. As previously mentioned, the double-blind study, despite its shortcomings, is the only reliable type of study when the protocol has been set up for a statistical evaluation.

For a discussion of therapeutic efficacy and toxicity, drugs useful in the treatment of depression may be divided into monoamine oxidase (MAO) inhibitors (hydrazine and non-hydrazine compounds) and non-MAO inhibitors.

MAO Inhibitors

The hydrazine compounds, such as Marplan®, Nardil®, and Niamid®, are all potentially capable of producing hepatocellular damage, as differentiated from the obstructive cholangiolitic type that occurs with the phenothiazines and their derivatives. The atropine-like effects such as blurring of vision, and atonic bladder and bowel are similar to those previously described with Thorazine. These minor side effects, as well as the occurrence of those cases of orthostatic hypotension, can usually be controlled by a reduction in dosage. The therapeutic efficacy of these drugs is still open to question.

In a study conducted at the Boston Psychopathic Hospital by Greenblatt and his associates, no significant therapeutic difference was noted in Marplan, Nardil (MAO inhibitor), and Tofranil® (non-MAO inhibitor) (11). EST was superior to these three forms of treatment in patients with the target symptom of depression. In view of the questionable therapeutic efficacy and potential toxicity of the hydrazine group, the pharmaceutical firms have been prompted to investigate other chemical series with MAO properties.

Parnate® is a nonhydrazine MAO inhibitor. Psychomotor stimulation and orthostatic hypotension may occur as in the hydrazine group. In addition, the familiar side effect of paradoxical hypertension has been reported with this compound, particularly in association with the ingestion of cheeses. At the present time, it is recommended that this medication be used only in an inpatient service or under very careful medical supervision (10 mg b.i.d. to 10 mg t.i.d.).

Non-MAO Inhibitors

Tofranil (25 mg b.i.d. to 25 mg q.i.d.) and Elavil® (25 mg t.i.d. to 50 mg t.i.d.) are the two most widely used agents in this group of compounds. Both are phenothiazine derivatives, and have the same potential toxicity and side effects of the parent compounds except for one important difference. These drugs do not potentiate narcotics or anaesthetic agents despite their chemical derivation. Otherwise, the contraindications in clinical management of side effects are the same for both groups of compounds. Norpramin®, a Tofranil derivative, was recently evaluated in the Tulane drug research program. Under double-blind conditions with a maximum dosage of 150 mg daily, it was clearly shown that this medication is significantly superior to placebo in patients with the target symptom of depression. It was also observed that the onset of therapeutic activity occurred during the first week of drug administration, a more rapid effect than noted with Tofranil. This observation is not surprising since the compound is an intermediate metabolite of Tofranil. However, the results of this study have not yet been fully confirmed by other investigators.

In Wittenborn's definitive evaluation in ninety-six depressed female patients, he found some significance existing between symptom clusters and responses to specific types of treatment (12). With Iproniazid®, he found that the symptoms of anxiety were lessened, as well as a reduction in the intensity of depression and phobias. Improved performance on the psychologic tests was observed. The patient saw himself as more friendly and less jittery. With Tofranil, only a significant reduction of the phobic symptomatology was seen. With electroconvulsive treatment, both anxiety and depression were significantly reduced. Self-perception was also improved. Some interesting cluster symptom results were: an adverse response to Tofranil was noted in patients with dependent self-critical personalities or histories of suicide attempts. If this group were excluded in the final results, then Tofranil would be superior to placebo in reducing anxiety. The anxious, angry, paranoid depressives improved on Tofranil, Iproniazid, and electroconvulsive treatment. Tofranil benefited the withdrawn, apathetic, depressed patient. It is interesting to note that Tofranil has been reported to increase the "hostility outward scores" which is an indication of the patient's ability to express anger in a more appropriate manner. It should be emphasized that any medication, no matter how efficacious, can never treat the underlying etiologic personality disorder that leads to the depression. In a similar manner, it should also be stressed that different approaches in psychotherapy technics must be applied to patients with different types of depressive syndromes.

The use of one MAO inhibitor with another MAO inhibitor is specifically contraindicated. As has been noted with the phenothiazines, a synergistic atropine-like effect may ensue with tremors, dry skin, and temperature elevation, sometimes resulting in convulsions, coma and death. Barbiturates should not be employed in treating such reactions because the central nervous system depression will be potentiated. If it is necessary to change antidepressive medications, the physician should allow at least an interval of one week before initiating the second drug. During this period, a mild tranquilizer could be given with safety.

ANTIANXIETY COMPOUNDS

The commercially available antianxiety compounds are too numerous and their structural formulas too varied to be presented in a logical manner. The discussion of these agents will thus be limited to the two most well-known compounds, Librium® (usual dosage varies from 10 mg b.i.d. to 25 mg q.i.d.) and Equanil® or Miltown® (200 mg q.i.d. to 400 mg q.i.d.). Drowsiness and ataxia are two of the most frequent side effects of Librium. Elderly patients are particularly susceptible to the development of ataxia with resulting accidents and injury. Small doses should be used in these patients. Sudden episodes of sleep have occurred in some patients while driving cars. Addiction accompanied by withdrawal seizures has occurred with doses above 200 mg daily. Meprobamate® has similar side effects, but the dose required to produce ataxia is usually well above the sedation threshold. Occasional physiological addiction has been reported on doses as low as 3200 mg daily.

The existence of cluster symptom groups within the anxiety-neurotic syndrome has not yet been adequately demonstrated in contrast to Wittenborn's finding in the depressive syndrome. Thus, there are some studies which show that these antianxiety agents have no clearly greater therapeutic efficacy than placebo. However, there is no doubt that these drugs are active compounds and that further evaluation of certain cluster groups within the anxiety syndrome will reveal these mild tranquilizers to have definite therapeutic efficacy in certain patient groups.

In one double-blind study, it has been shown that phenobarbital, grs ¼ q.i.d., approaches the therapeutic efficacy of Equanil or Miltown in the treatment of the anxiety syndrome. It is my opinion that phenobarbital and the other minor tranquilizers should be prescribed for anxiety neurosis if the patient's symptomatology is severely interfering with his ability to function in his environment as well as with his ability to relate to the physician. It should not be necessary to resort to the major tranquilizers such as the phenothiazines since their toxicity and side effects far outweigh their therapeutic efficacy in the nonpsychotic patient.

Since side effects of the minor tranquilizers are mild compared to the major tranquilizers, there is a tendency to use these drugs in a careless manner. The mild sedative effects of these medications can result in serious accidents if inquiries are not made into the patient's routine activities. The patient should be particularly cautioned not to drive during the first two to three days of medication or for several days following an increase in dosage of any of these agents if sedative or ataxic side effects are anticipated.

ALCOHOLISM

It has been suggested that the phenothiazines (particularly the dimethyl subgroup which includes Thorazine) have no definite place in the treatment of alcoholism. Since Thorazine mildly inhibits the breakdown of alcohol and definitely potentiates the narcotic effects of alcohol, it has been considered by many physicians that these phenothiazine agents are too dangerous to be used in a routine manner with the alcoholic patient (14). In addition, episodes of severe orthostatic hypotension can occur in the alcoholic patient when he is administered phenothiazine drugs. Since it has been noted by Sharpey-Schafer and others that the mild peripheral neuropathy of the alcoholic patient can have an inhibitory effect on the baroceptor reflexes, further inhibition of these reflexes by the phenothiazine drugs can result in a severe episode of orthostatic hypotension in this type of patient (15). While Librium has assumed a more important place in the management of the acute alcoholic syndrome of delirium tremens as well as in the treatment of the chronic alcoholic with anxiety, paraldehyde may still have a place in the treatment of delirium tremens. Neither Thorazine nor Librium has been shown to have clearly superior therapeutic efficacy to paraldehyde in the treatment of this acute alcoholic syndrome.

Since the alcoholic patient has frequent depressive reactions, combinations of small dosages of a minor tranquilizer with mild dosages of an antidepressant non-MAO inhibitor are sometimes indicated for the chronic alcoholic during the initial phase of his sobriety.

SUMMARY

Psychopharmacologic treatment can produce gratifying results, and well controlled drug investigations leave no doubt as to the effectiveness of some of these compounds. The inconvenience of most side effects is negligible when weighed against the distress of the seriously ill patient. However, the knowledge of the biochemical effects of these drugs is still in its infancy, particularly regarding toxicity and side effects. Since all of these psychopharmacologic agents pass the maternal-fetal placental barrier, extreme discretion is urged regarding the use of these agents during pregnancy until more adequate animal and human data are available (4). The risks involved with the use of psychopharmacologic drugs must be carefully considered, particularly before they are administered to the less seriously ill patient.

REFERENCES

1. Haas, H., Fink, H., and Hartfelder, G.: The placebo problem. *Psychopharmacol Serv. Cent. Bull.*, 2:1-65, 1965.
2. Honigfeld, G.: Nonspecific factors in treatment. *Dis. Nerv. Syst.*, 25:145-156 and 225-239, 1964.

3. Shapiro, R. K.: Etiological factors in placebo effect. *J.A.M.A.*, *187*:136-138, 1964.

4. Gallant, D. M.: Clinical management of side effects and toxicity in Psychopharmacologic Therapy. *Bull. Tulane Med. Fac.*, 2:179-186, 1963.

5. Katz, M. M., and Cole, J. O.: Research conference on drugs and community care: A review and analysis. *Psychopharmacol Serv. Cent. Bull.*, 1-13, 1961.

6. Cole, J. O., *et al.*: Phenothiazine treatment in acute schizophrenia. *Arch. Gen. Psychiat.*, *10*:246-261, 1964.

7. Goldberg, S.: Paper presented at the American College of Neuropsychopharmacology Meeting in Wash., D. C., October, 1964.

8. Gallant, D. M., Bishop, M. P., Timmons, E., and Steele, C. A.: A controlled evaluation of trifluperidol: A new potent psychopharmacologic agent. *Curr. Ther. Res.*, 5:463-471.

9. Bishop, M. P., and Gallant, D. M.: Trifluperidol in paranoid and non-paranoid schizophrenics. *Curr. Ther. Res.*, 7:96-102, 1965.

10. Hoyles, Fred: *Of Men and Galaxies.* Univ. of Wash. Press, 1964.

11. Greenblatt, Milton, Grosser, G. H., and Wechsler, Henry: A comparative study of selected antidepressant medications and EST, *119*:144-153, 1962.

12. Wittenborn, J. R.: Paper presented at the American College of Neuropsychopharmacology Meeting in Wash., D. C., January, 1965.

13. Hollister, Leo: Lecture presented at Tulane Dept. of Psychiatry, October, 1964.

14. Tipton, D. L., Jr., Sutherland, V. C., Burbridge, T. N., and Simon, A.: Effect of chlorpromazine on blood level of alcohol in rabbits. *Amer. J. Physiol.*, *200*:1007-1010, 1961.

15. Sharpey-Schafer, E. P.: Syncope. *Brit. Med. J.*, *1*:506-509, 1956.

PSYCHIATRIC EMERGENCIES IN
MEDICAL PRACTICE

ARTHUR P. BURDON, M.D.

T HE FAMILY PHYSICIAN often feels unduly threatened by a call for help in a psychiatric emergency. As calmly professional as he is in medical or surgical crises, the physician may be unprepared to cope with the onslaught of fearful anxiety in the patient and the immediate family in an emotional storm. The worried practitioner may well learn from an organization famed for its cool work in stormy emergencies of another sort—the U. S. Coast Guard—whose motto "Semper Paratus," expresses a useful philosophy. This paper is written in such a spirit.

Psychiatric emergencies may be placed in five categories for convenience of discussion: (1) acute severe anxiety (panic); (2) acute severe agitation with or without depression; (3) acute psychotic confusion (manic-depressive or schizophrenia); (4) acute severe suicidal behavior or ideation, and (5) acute toxic delerium. In these groups there are patients who are severely disturbed in the emergency situation, yet who may not have other problems, while there are others whose life situation is one of great chronic travail as well. The important consideration for the medical practitioner in handling the emergency is the degree and type of panicky anxiety connected with any of these phenomena, whether in the patient or in the family, in the staff of the hospital emergency unit or in the physician himself.

Psychiatric emergencies are a combination of *fear* and *family* in all respects, the appropriate management of these emergencies involves adequate handling of anxiety in all persons involved in the emergency crisis. Psychiatric emergencies do not represent

173

a certain severity of psychiatric disease itself. Indeed, there are emergencies in which there is very little physical or emotional disease in any member of the family except a momentary reactive panic, such as that which might occur after the first Mittlesmertz in an immature and anxious girl away from home at college. Other psychiatric emergencies may represent emotional conditions and indicate the raw edge of complete psychosis. Thus, a delirium tremens in which the patient is totally disoriented as to time, place, and person and in which he sees and fears violent hallucinatory objects and persons, represents a toxic situation in which the patients rational mind is totally in abeyance because of the poisoning of the alcohol.

Perhaps the most common form of psychiatric emergency is the "family fight." Here two markedly immature people have gotten into a violent argument and there is build up of unpleasant feelings regarding each other, all too frequently over trivial matters. Helped on by alcohol, drugs, fatigue or other family matters and crises, the husband and wife may become so severely enraged and troubled with each other as to precipitate physical and emotional conditions in themselves requiring medical assistance. Many acute heart attacks may be traced to severe emotional upsets around family quarrels, as indeed can attacks of asthma, paroxysmal tachycardia, acute colitis and other psychosomatic reactive conditions. The medical practitioner should be alert for acute emotional crises as the precipitating event in any psychosomatic situation.

Patients who represent psychiatric emergencies in office practice will often be psychotic or in a very disturbed neurotic state. While these neurotic patients are less ill in the long run, the immediate emergency crisis may be very dangerous or traumatic. Thus an attempted suicide by a neurotic may be only a gesture of attention-getting or hostility. Yet the family reaction may provoke the angry patient into further and more serious suicidal impulsiveness if he is not responded to in a loving and compassionate manner by the family. Physicians may be called for home visits on account of hysterical fainting spells, immature temper tantrums, and family quarrels much more often than for major psychiatric diseases. Hysterical murderous rages, self mutilation, or murderous hostility towards others as a result of alcoholism in an impulsive immature personality constitute a significant but small number of psychiatric emergencies.

The psychotic patients most often seen as emergencies are the severely depressed reactions or the acute schizophrenic withdrawals or excitements. The depressed patient may be either totally withdrawn or agitated. If withdrawn, the patient usually does not eat or sleep well and may have delusions of guilt. He moans repetitively about his sins of the past or the present and repeats his great yearning for some release from this piteous condition, often by suicide. The agitated depressive is seen pacing the floor and unable to sit still while wringing his hands and picking at his face, arms, and clothing. The agitation is clear in the voice, in the manner and in the desperate look in the eye of these patients who see themselves as on the brink of being overwhelmed by acute and painful unmitigated panic. Their fear is of inner drives overwhelming them and they are unable to sleep. Without question these two types of psychotic depressions require immediate hospitalization and psychiatric treatment. Yet the family physician's job is not over—he more than anyone else, should be able to support the anxious, tense, and difficult feelings of the family. In fact, the physician's skillful and tactful handling of a referral to a psychiatrist will make important and major contributions towards the future medical well being and emotional well being of this family in relation to the family doctor. First of all, the patient is much more likely to go to and stay in the hospital with the proper attitude towards treatment if he and his family are handled right. He is also much more likely to return gratefully to the family physician's care thereafter.

Unrecognized depression still represents the chief psychiatric disorder in general medicine and represents the acute threat of suicide in certain emergency situations. Even with hospitalized patients, one must recognize the risk in older patients of depressive reactions, particularly in convalescence from serious disease, coronary thrombosis or cerebral vascular accident. Many of the patients become severely depressed in a quiet desperation, which too often escapes the notice of the busy physician. Reserpine, used to treat hypertension, may precipitate an acute depression.

Patients whose diagnosis is of terminal cancer may impulsively attempt suicide or show undue emotional reactions of many sorts including many distorted guilt reactions and preoccupations with unrealistic desires for medical interventions. These patients need active and self conscious cooperation between themselves and their physician and their families in order to bear the pain and anxiety of approaching death. In the hospital treatment of the chronically ill, elderly, or seriously ill patient it is advisable that their nurses and their family, as well as the attending physician monitor the emotional state of their patients at all times. In no instance should a seriously depressed patient go without psychiatric referral.

Insomnia, anorexia, loss of interest and drive, a depressive or self punitive mood, and a sharp change in the patient's attitude towards the future and his hopefulness about the future are sufficient clinical signs to lead the physician to inquire further into the patient's mental status and not to accept a simply denial on the part of the patient as an explanation. It is important to remember that patients who are seriously ill use denial, distortion, and projection as mechanisms to dull the psychic pain of fearful ideas about their fate—this makes the physician's responsibility in determining the need for psychiatric referral grave indeed.

Among the schizophrenic patients likely to be seen in an emergency are those who go into an excited catatonic state—those who run about wildly and whose conversation is irrelevant and tangential and whose speech and attitude indicate their complete disconnection with the world of reality. These patients are irresponsible and sometimes dangerous in their behavior. They should be handled so that they can be given intramuscular medication and quieted and immediately hospitalized. Paranoid psychotic patients who are assaultive, hostile and often dangerous may threaten their family or neighbors with deadly weapons in an acute crescendo of fearful anxiety against the supposed harm that is being done by these very friends and neighbors.

Acute schizophrenic illnesses often begin by sudden changes in behavior and personality of the patient, a broken sleep pattern with odd behavior at night is a signal of serious disturbance. Common symptoms are delusions of infidelity or of persecution on the part of husband and wife for each other. Without sufficient proof and with only the vagueness of suspicion and resentfulness, many patients mount enormous rages at their spouses or other members of their families for alleged persecution or embarrassments. When called into such a situation, the physician will obviously not argue the reality of the contentions of the patient, but will attempt to win the patient's confidence by a calm medical approach to the patient's acute anxiety regardless of its rational or irrational source. The patient may accept mental hospitalization and medication for acute anxiety or tension over their family problems, without the physician being committed to a value judgment as to the reality of the patient's view of the preoccupying family problem. Later the physician will check the objective truth of the patient's allegations and will look for other evidence of paranoid thinking and schizophrenic reactions.

Acute brain syndromes can be associated with any illness that might produce high fever, a disturbance of metabolism, or a state of exhaustion. Acute brain syndromes are characterized by excitement and fearful hallucinations, disorientation as to time, place, and person and confusion as to motivations, purposes, and intent. Often these hallucinations are visual, sometimes tactile and auditory. Acute brain syndromes as a result of alcoholism are well known in the state of delirium tremens. Similar acute brain syndromes have been recorded as a consequence of drug addiction, barbiturate addiction, or toxic reactions to the use of drugs which are incompatible with one another.

Other conditions which may present psychiatric emergencies are organic in origin. Certain hyperthyroid patients may show acute excitability, irritability and restlessness with or without paranoid features in the mental status. Certain diabetics who are suffering from hyperinsulism show marked tension and difficulty in orientation and sweating as if they were suffering a toxic brain syndrome. Certain post partum and post surgical reactions are psychotic in nature and usually show a toxic picture with either schizophrenic or depressive manifestations. Often these phenomena represent disturbances of metabolism, as well as of psychic equilibrium. It is well to remember that many patients react to the enforced regression of surgery and of the anesthetic by tremendous emotional upheaval as well as by the physical trauma associated with the surgery.

As has been stated before, psychiatric emergencies are a combination of *fear* and panic, whether reacted to psychotically or neurotically, and the *family* reacts with their own coping defenses. The management of psychiatric emergencies should be psychotherapeutic, and not the result of impulsive action induced in some physicians by the manifest anxiety of the patient, the family, the staff, or the physician's personal reactions. It is most important for us to bear in mind that anxiety, particularly acute and severe anxiety, is one of the most contagious conditions known. It can clearly be transferred to those around the patient. The physician is a professional and his task is not to avoid anxiety in himself or in others but to listen attentively to what is said and to understand as fully as possible the source of the acute tension and anxiety in the family and in the patient. The patient wants and needs direct intervention but his greatest need is for a physician who is alert to the misunderstandings, exaggerations, painful contradictions, omissions, and other sudden impulsive emotional characteristics that color the acute emergency.

The most reassuring thing the physician can do is to "Declare the past, diagnose the present, foretell the future: and practice these arts effectively—to help, or at least to do no harm." These words are quoted from Hippocrates, whose further comments on the reassuring value of a physician also bear repeating, "For some patients, though conscious that their condition is perilous, recover their health simply through their contentment with the goodness of the physician." The basic premise of psychotherapy of any kind, namely basic positive empathy, is facilitated through the willingness of the physician to accept and to bear the brunt unblinkingly of all the excited emotionality, vicious ideation, threats, tears, hallucinations, or whatever else may come from the patient, in a calm and rational way. The key to the physician's success with acute psychiatric emergencies then is his own ability to tolerate anxiety in himself and others and not to react defensively or emotionally on his own part.

This equanimity on the part of the physician has an enormous calming effect on the upset patient and family in most circumstances, even in drug delirias or psychoses which seemingly have rendered the patient fairly imperceptive of the doctor's presence. The appearance of the doctor then begins the active intervention of bringing rational thought to the problem at hand. The physician must proceed with the job, as outlined by Hippocrates, to make his examination and to be thoroughly and calmly busy with his job of taking a history and doing a physical examination through to completion. The length of time and manner in which the physician does this careful examination will determine in most instances the kind of response that the family will have to his therapy.

The doctor should be aware not to delegate his responsibilities for his supportive role, even though he may be out of his depth from a strictly medical point of view. It is much more advisable for the patient to be referred to a psychiatrist as a consultant than to be dumped into a strange specialist's office with all familiar supportive relationships with the family physician being removed. It is not surprising that such patients do feel that they have been rejected and develop a negative attitude not only towards the psychiatrist to whom they were referred but towards their family physician as well. It is quite common for such patients to view their acute emergency as having been an imposition on their family physician.

It may be that the accusation about psychiatry as being a defender of the status quo and a profession which attempts to achieve social adjustment even at great personal inner price of inner freedom, would have justification if this be the common pattern of referral to a psychiatrist. There are too many instances in which the over-wrought excited patient is the only reasonable one in the situation and the family, having scapegoated the patient, is calling in the physician to add the coup de grâce to their execution of the patient's personal liberties and inner freedom. One constantly must beware of the family which does this to their weaker members. One is aware of this occurring commonly in teenage youth and children when their parents act out their difficulties by condemning their children who, responding to the inner tensions of the family, break down because of the weakness of their ego defenses. One perhaps is less familiar with the fact that this same scapegoating mechanism occurs in the elderly members of the family as well.

One of the common misapprehensions in handling patients is whether or not the physician should be frank with the patient about his need for hospitalization and commitment for mental observation. Skirmishes are going on sporadically between certain physicians and psychiatrists on the subject. Psychiatrists are firmly convinced that the patient should never be tricked or lied to, that he should be confronted directly with the physician's good intentions and honest motives in hospitalizing the patient who is already intensely and highly suspicious. The physician not only must act trustworthy but also be trustworthy.

One misapprehension is that the usual psychiatric emergency patient is as *violent in actions* and outcomes as he is in speech or in emotionality. This is certainly not true. For all disturbed patients who have become violent, there are many many hundreds of patients equally or more seriously disturbed who are very tractable to personal or physical handling. One other misconception is with regard to the discussing of hostility, aggression or suicidal ideation openly and directly with the patient. Many physicians regard this as a tabooed area and hold back for fear of insulting the patient or in some way making the emotional condition worse. But it cannot be emphasized too strongly that forthright inquiry into all appropriate areas of the patient's attitudes in life is in order. The patient usually responds to direct inquiries by giving appropriate and often full explanations of their behavior. This provides considerable sense of relief that someone now is willing to listen to them talk about forbidden subjects. To discuss suicide with a depressed patient is not only in order but very helpful.

The best safeguard against misunderstanding of the meaning

of the psychiatric emergency is to take an adequate history and to ask questions, remembering people in acute emergencies have not got the defenses that they usually have, and are more likely to tell the unvarnished truth. It is extremely important to get the patient's view of what the difficulty is, then to compare it with the responsible other members of the family and to inquire further to reach some consensus of opinions so that a rational approach can be reached to decide the issues at hand. An accurate history of the present illness and of the genesis of the acute emergency is most beneficial to help outline the difficulty to the consulting psychiatrist as well as to understand it for the family physician himself. It is often true that functional psychosis starts as a response to specific traumatic events which are soon forgotten if not recalled within a short time of onset of their illness.

The patient expects and should get as specific a diagnosis and prognosis as possible. In addition he should receive reassurance and treatment for the acute overwhelming anxiety either in himself or the members of his family. Thus some patients should receive immediate doses of barbiturates or tranquilizers intramuscularly, other patients should be hospitalized away from their family, while other patients should be given an appointment to discuss alone at length their troubles on some future date, while other patients should be immediately supported in their difficulties with their families, and still other patients should be firmly confronted with their attempts at secondary gain through hysterical over-reaction. The important principle to bear in mind is that, once he knows the situation, the family physician should *go ahead actively* with immediate psychotherapeutic measures which he deems appropriate to the situation. *He must act.* He can prohibit, permit, help to express, order, reassure, manipulate the environment, hospitalize, or ignore as he sees suitable to the situation.

These techniques, sometimes called confrontation techniques, are most effective in the midst of the crisis situation. Recent theory about the effects of psychotherapy have indicated that the patient's response to a word, an action, or an attitude of a physician during the time of an acute severe emotional crisis can be more lasting, more effective, and more crucially influential in the path the patient follows in his future life than any blandishments from parents or psychiatrists during states of relative tranquility and inertia in the mental apparatus. Thus the crisis situation should be explored with vigor and in detail. The patient should be helped to label, reconceptualize, and reflect on his crisis experience and to learn from it something more about his difficulties.

In some acute family tension states and with great anxiety and hostility between members of the family, the overwhelmed patient may be able to use a hospital in the old fashioned sense of the word as a "retreat.' Psychiatric "crisis wards" have been proposed and used in hospitals for allowing a temporary regression for the distressed patient. He is able to withdraw from the life-impasse in order to regroup his ego forces and to begin to react again in a more rational manner to their problems. Voluntary admission for two to three weeks to these wards have dramatically reduced the percentage of patients whose acute onset of emotional disturbance would have led on to state mental hospitalization if not handled immediately. The old principle of "splinting them where they lie" is valid in psychiatry as well as it is in orthopedic surgery.

I do not advise *referral to* a psychiatrist as a reaction to a psychiatric emergency, but *active consultation with* the psychiatrist either in person or by telephone. It it important for the family physician to have on hand several friends in the profession of psychiatry who know him well in and out of anxiety situations, and who are willing to listen to him describe the emergency situation and give him their frank and honest opinion when the physician needs consultation. Thus, one should *be fully prepared* for psychiatric emergencies. Preparation and adequate positive Doctor-Patient relationships with the patients tend to prevent the occurrence of unexpected psychiatric emergencies in a stable practice population. Nevertheless emergencies will occur. It is wise to be fully prepared for an emergency by thinking out what plans, what hospital, what medication one would use in advance. Thus the treatment action is planned by choice and does not evolve as an expedient adjustment to necessity in a situation without adequate resources and without imagination or forethought, a situation in which the anxiety and defenses of the family and even the physician and hospital staff may be at the lowest ebb.

Preparation for the emergency should involve the use of certain hospital beds for crisis admission, the use of intramuscular sedatives, or tranquilizers to immediately control untoward actions or ideas, and the availability of suitable physical protection both for the patient and for others during the examination and early treatment of the patient. Often troublesome have been house calls for acutely disturbed schizophrenic patients who have barricaded themselves in their rooms and who are otherwise totally resistive to persuasion and who must be handled by physical force. It is often the physician's misfortune not to have known this obvious fact in advance of his visit, and for the family not to have called in adequate help. It is important to remember the availability and the appropriateness of the police for any patient who is disturbing others and who will not respond to persuasion. Parenthetically it is important to remember that most paranoid and agitated psychotic patients can still have presence of mind enough to calm down in the presence of four or five husky men who intend to collar them if they do not calm down. Many disturbed patients will become quiet under such circumstances without having been touched by the attending personnel.

A problem of enormous frustration is that of seeking an emergency hospital bed for an acutely disturbed patient, who may not require prolonged mental hospitalization and whose family may object to mental hospitalization under any conditions. It is thus most fortuitous that in New Orleans and in more and more communities around the country there are psychiatric wards and facilities for acute treatment of emergency emotional states in the general hospital with neither stigma or difficulties in admission. One would hope that these liberal conditions would extend to the alcoholic as well. They do in our community but this is not universally true.

As to drug management of the hyperactive or over-excited or assaultive patient, my recommendation is that adequate medication in a single dose be given rather than mild repeated doses. It is often noted that the patient fights inadequate doses and becomes more disturbed as their consciousness is dimmed by a small dose of tranquilizer or barbiturates. It is particularly true of manic patients or severely excited paranoid psychotic patients that they may tolerate extreme doses of tranquilizers and barbiturates without going to sleep. It is advisable to start with heavy doses of chlorpromazine intramuscularly (between 50 and 150 mgms) or to use 7½ grains of sodium amytal (I.M.) for tranquilization of these patients. There is rarely ever any occasion in the immediate situation where other drugs will be necessary.

Many physicians make errors in medication with their psychiatric problems. A common error is the giving of sedatives or tranquilizers to patients with histories of suicidal attempts or ruminations. Other mistakes include the use of mild tranquilizers, or inadequate doses of drugs, such as meprobamate and chlordiazepoxide, in schizophrenia. Such misjudgments result from either incorrect diagnosis or lack of understanding of indications for different groups of psychiatric drugs. As a simple rule of thumb, the family physician may well learn the use of one antischizophrenic and anti-excitement drug, preferrably chlorpromazine. Combined with barbiturates, with which the family doctor is already familiar, chlorpromazine should be adequate for the handling of any psychiatric emergency. In cases of depression sufficient to alarm the family, I suggest psychiatric consultation immediately and dosages of medication or electric shock as indicated by the psychiatrist. I would not favor the prescription of anti-depressive medication and the use of such medication by the patient without psychiatric consultation.

Physicians occasionally prescribe potentially lethal combinations of antidepressants, such as a non-monoamine-oxidase inhibitor with or shortly after use of the monoamine- oxidase inhibitor. This results in a toxic state in many patients. Other drugs are sometimes erroneously given for psychiatric conditions. Amphetamines in the schizophrenic and seriously emotionally unstable person may be quite disruptive. Thyroid medication in the depressive patient may mobilize him to suicidal acting out; similarly amphetamines are contraindicated in the obese borderline psychotic patient. Narcotics are not to be used, of course, in psychophysiological reactions or personality disorders if they can possibly be avoided. The use of female or male hormones in other than specific menopausal reactions is to be abjurred, particularly in schizophrenic or in severe depressive reactions.

SUMMARY

In handling psychiatric emergencies various recommendations are made concerning the approach, diagnosis, psychotherapeutic, drug and hospital management. Psychiatric emergencies have been described as acute ego defective states in which there has been a break down in the handling of fear (severe anxiety) and family in patients with varying emotional conditions all the way from mild neurotic and immature reactions to acute paranoid homicidal schizophrenics.

In these emergencies the physician is advised to do an adequate physical and psychiatric examination both of the patient alone and of the patient with the relatives in attendance, and to make as informed a decision regarding the handling of the patient as he is capable of doing. If it is necessary for psychiatric consultation, this should be done immediately in person or by telephone with a confrere whose opinion and judgment is known from previous contacts. The consultation can be helpful in suggesting immediate hospitalization or referral for psychiatric treatment, or other psychotherapeutic measures.

The aim is to restore control of the patient's impulses by doing something appropriate and meaningful which will improve his controls. The most important single element is to conquer the fear and anxiety in the situation and to be prepared in advance for handling the patients through adequate knowledge of acute psychiatric emergencies.

THE MENOPAUSE AND ITS MANAGEMENT

ERNEST O. SVENSON, M.D.

THE MENOPAUSE IS a complex period, a normal process in the
life cycle that lends itself to pathological formations both in the
organic and psychological areas. It is a time of organic change,
and a time of psychological reckoning: a time when bodily
changes force recognition of aging, when the culturally idealized
youthful aspirations cannot be maintained, and when the woman
must come to an individual resolution of the fact that she can no
longer bear children. Thus an area of fantasy is blocked; no
longer can she feel that her problems can be solved by another
child or starting a new family. Her very identity is threatened
and she must determine in some way her place in society, lacking
her child-bearing potential. This is a true loss, and thus the most
frequent form of reaction is some type of depression or depressive
equivalent.

The organic processes, though varying a great deal in onset
and duration, certainly are well understood. The decrease in
ovarian function and hormonal changes leading to menstrual
irregularities and cessation, bodily changes in distribution of
fat, etc. are well known. Other symptoms are certainly more
difficult to evaluate because of their wide variation. Vasomotor
instability, hot flushes, palpitations, and vertigo are common and
the response to hormonal replacement therapy is usually good.
However, at the other end of the spectrum, the psychic symptoms,
such as irritability, anxiety, depression, and mood swings, respond
much less favorably. Thus, the psychological correllates of the
menopause seem to respond poorly to physiological replacement
of the lacking hormones. It would follow that there is emotional

stress at a different level than that of pure physiology. Indeed, at other times when there are large hormonal changes, puberty and pregnancy, psychological symptoms are less frequent and severe than during the climacterium. This would seem to indicate that it is a period of psychological stress and reaction produced and enhanced by organic changes but having its own psychological meanings with antecedents in the past developmental patterns and adaptations of the individual. The symptoms and outcome will then be largely determined by the individual's past success in developing her true sexual and maternal identifications, and the flexibility of her adjustment capabilities. This period, I believe, is the last great developmental stage, or identity crisis of the individual. In men, the physiological correllates are not as definite, but, nonetheless, a corresponding redefinition of self must be confirmed.

Medical literature is replete with thousands of articles on the endocrinological and gynecological aspects of the menopause. However, relatively few purely psychological studies have been done. I would like to briefly summarize some of the extensive work done by Therese Benedek (1) in attempting to correllate the two areas of investigation. A number of women undergoing psychoanalysis by different analysts, took daily vaginal smears to determine the phase of their menstrual cycle. The slides were read by an independent group, and from the analytic material predictions were made as to the phase of the menstrual cycle. The data was then compared and the correllation was extremely accurate, leading them to postulate that there are psychological patterns during the menstrual cycle depending on the predominate hormone. During the ovulatory, or estrogen phase, the woman is more extroverted and her heterosexual desires increase until the time of ovulation. After this, during the progesterone phase, the woman's interest turns more inward toward herself and children, and finally, in the premenstrual phase of hormonal decline, she is more anxious, aggressive, dependent and demanding. This would then explain the emotional difficulties during the menopause as being at least partially due to the decrease in hormone production, in other words, somewhat comparable to the premenstrual phase of the menstrual cycle. Consequently in the beginning menopause, as in the premenstrual phase, when the hormonal levels are low, the woman is often tense, cranky, hostile and resentful or depressed, feels deprecated, and is more dependent and demanding. Normally these premenstrual symptoms decrease with the progress of psychosexual maturation, that is pregnancy, motherhood and a satisfactory sexual life. There is, in effect, a developmental absorption of some of the stresses responsible for the premenstrual tension, both in the psychological and physiological spheres, if the woman obtains full feminine maturation maternally and sexually. There are some women, however, whose early psychosexual development causes rebellion against or retards and inhibits the satisfaction of the normal feminine wishes. These women often continue to suffer severely from premenstrual tension or depression and frequently have a very difficult menopause.

Most women have symptoms during the climacterium but they are usually not severe enough to interfere with their daily routines. About fifteen per cent of women have severe disturbances during this period. In this group the menopause did not seem to be the only cause of difficulty, for most had emotional problems far anteceding the menopause. In fact, though most wanted to blame organic factors, they honestly believed they were of a psychogenic nature (2). What, then, makes this a particularly difficult time for some women, especially when fears of pregnancy and discomfort of menstruation (indeed oftentimes called "the curse") cease to exist? Some of the fears seem culturally determined. Our culture places great value on youth and a rather flambouyant pseudo-sexuality and tends to fear age and relegate it to an inferior status. Thus, with the decrease in sexual function and physical changes, the woman often takes it as a severe blow to her ego and fears that she will become valueless. Of greater importance, however, is the past emotional development of the woman. If a female has had a secure early development during which she could identify with a mother who is happy and confident in her own feminine role, and a stable father with whom to relate, she has a very good chance of passing through further maturation successfully. Normally, the woman marries, bears children and derives meaningful gratification in her feminine role as wife and mother; i.e., sexually and reproductively. This woman should tolerate the menopause well. She may be bothered by vaso-vegetative symptoms, mood swings, and minor depressive reactions, but she will continue to function well. Freed from the major tensions of sexuality and from the time consuming tasks of child care, increased energy is available for increasing her scope of interests in community and cultural activities. Her relationship with her husband may become enriched, the marriage more tranquil, and sex, though less frequent, fully as enjoyable as before. Her love becomes less ambivalent and jealous and she is more tolerant. The relationship with her grandchildren may be more tender, less demanding, and freer from conflict than even the mother's love may be.

The climacterium is thus a true developmental phase, in which a new integration is reached and psychic energy redirected along new lines of adaptation. I feel, therefore, it is much more than just a time of defensive reaction to sexual loss. Her former reproductivity may be channeled along artistic lines, her maternal feelings into wider social activities. It is a period in which the emotional needs are desexualized, releasing psychic energy for sublimation and further integration of the personality. As during any time of stress, there is a tendency toward regression during the menopause. A common regression that most women experience to a degree is depression. The loss is a very real one— sexuality in many of its ramifications, and is experienced as a narcissistic blow. All that was gained at puberty is undergoing dissolution and leaves her feeling greatly devalued. Culturally, this sense of loss is reinforced, for in America age does not carry with it the respect that some societies give it. The most common type of depression is somewhat different from the usual endogenous depression. Mood is much more fluctuating, self-accusation is less persistent, and there is more self pity and open aggressiveness. She tends to describe her sufferings in superlatives; there is much bodily preoccupation and she often feels she is being inadequately treated. There are also depressions that reach psychotic proportions, and in these the possibility of suicide must always be considered.

Denial is another defense used to avoid the reality of the menopause. The woman may become hypomanic in her attempt to prove nothing has changed. Frequently, sex will be overstressed in dress and activities. She may act coquetishly adolescent, or even become vulgar in her sexual openness; she may give up her old circle of friends and join much younger groups, often very socially inferior, and may become sexually promiscuous. Although transient and controlled episodes of increased sexual needs are common during this period, the bizarreness and persistence of this behavior indicates pathology. It is very difficult to treat this type of behavior, for any indication that the activity is inappropriate is met with strong denial and anger. When the defense fails, a severe depression is apt to occur. Treatment should be cautious with an attempt to rechannel the energy into more acceptable modes. Hypochondriasis is another common manifestation. Extreme preoccupation with any part of the body can occur, but frequently the genitals are involved, with fears of malignancy, indicating the great underlying fear of the sexual loss. The actual hormonal changes, with the corresponding vasovegetative symptoms, enhance the bodily preoccupations and fear, further increasing anxiety, which may exaggerate the symptoms, creating a vicious cycle of ever increasing intensity. Hormones may be of value, with firm reassurance and an attempt to redirect attention to the external environment.

Withdrawal into a compulsive martyr type existence may be attempted by the patient to insulate herself from the change. Intense preoccupation with the children is common, either to foster their close ties of dependency on her, or to maintain the closeness by demanding complete care from them. This is usually a continuation of an old defense, based on early parental dependency that was never resolved. She may now use the children as a way to avoid facing the external world. The most intense involvement is most often with the sons, and she may become very jealous of, and angry at the daughter-in-law, who has become to her an unwelcomed competitor.

Psychoses are usually of the depressive type; however, paranoid reactions as well as mixtures of the two, occur. Marked changes in sexual responsiveness may be met with—formerly frigid women may become receptive and orgastic; frigidity may occur in previously responsive women. Phobias and compulsive ritualistic acts are not uncommon.

Sometimes the alleviations of anxiety by drugs is enough to allow the individual to tolerate the stress and to a lesser extent test out and adapt to new methods of action. However, all too often drugs merely promote withdrawal and decreased level of function without solving the underlying difficulties. They may make the patient easier to get along with because of less reactivity, but they do not promote individual internal well-being or positive conflict solution. Drugs are all too often a method used to avoid facing the anxiety within a patient that could best be resolved by bringing it into an interpersonal therapeutic relationship. They can become an antitherapeutic measure based on denial or rejection: "Take this medicine and get rid of your problem—do not bother me with it." Often the result is a patient who functions far below her potential because of the inhibiting side effects of the drugs, and the chronic depression is increased by the refusal of the doctor to help the patient face the psychological issues, making her feel all the more unacceptable. I am not advocating the dropping of psychotropic drugs—at times they can be very helpful—but I maintain that they can be much more effectively used in conjunction with a willingness to explore the conflicts of the patient.

You would be amazed at the effect of simply telling the patient, "No, I will not attempt to remove all your symptoms with drugs, but I will tell you what will be helpful for you to do; I will explain why you feel as you do, and be willing to explore the causes of your discomfort with you." Not only does this display your confidence in the patients' own abilities, but it gives her the knowledge that you will be supportive and willing to understand. This may be enough to cause the patient to actively attempt to master her problems. Anxiety is not always a "bad" symptom—to be removed completely; it can serve as a force to cause change. Supportive therapy does not mean placating or agreeing with the patient. Manipulative and unrealistic behavior should be pointed out, along with its adverse consequences. Anger should be openly dealt with and not avoided—this in itself can relieve some of the patient's anxious guilt. If the patient knows you are not rejecting of her hostility, you have a much better chance of becoming a trusted ally to whom she can turn for constructive advice, rather than a tool to be manipulated or a receptacle for endless complaints.

Short term therapy is often very effective. A forty-four-year-old woman, mother of four, when threatened by the menopause, changed from an open, aggressive, energetic woman into a rather withdrawn person whose only function was to please her husband's and her children's slightest whim. Fearing their loss, her wish to keep them interested and dependent on her had the effect of turning a previously well-run home into a chaotic place. The children, doing as they pleased, treated her as a maid; and her husband's attentiveness decreased. She was faced with the problem of suppressing an ever increasing rage at being used and ignored. She came to my office after having several episodes, for which she was amnesic, of smashing dishes and having to be bodily restrained from attacking members of the household. When she was able to verbalize her anger, her fears of loss of womanhood, of being deserted by her family once they felt her valueless, she was able to regain control of her household and become involved in community work. Although she would become more openly angry, she was easier to live with than the previous martyr.

Firm and direct advice can be valuable. If one sees a patient who formerly has been productive become withdrawn, depressed, inactive and filled with feelings of unworthiness, it is obvious that activity, greater participation, and perhaps the development of new interests are indicated. This is not obvious to the patient and often firm insistence that she follow your suggestions is enough to start her toward recovery. I often prescribe exercises in short term therapy. It is not only sound physiologically speaking, but it also indicates an actively constructive approach and utilizes the muscular system to discharge some of the pent-up anxiety. The same applies to other activities from handicrafts and gardening to organizational work or paid employment. The activity should fit the individual—a college graduate would probably not find making pot holders very ego gratifying.

In the treatment of somatic complaints, the doctor can unconsciously become an ally of the symptom, endowing it with much interest and importance in his attempt to treat it medically. This gratification of the defense will tend to perpetuate it. Thus the doctor can be a force against an escape into illness, or an unwitting reinforcement of the emotionally based symptom, which can lead to a chronically complaining invalid.

There is no set way to do psychotherapy; there are many differing effective approaches. Sometimes the marital relationship is strained by the hidden fears of both partners as they approach their fifties, and both must be seen. An example is that of a couple in their late forties. He, beginning to fear loss of sexual potency, began drinking excessively; she, fearing she was no longer sexually desirable (and drinking meant to her that he was chasing other women) became increasingly moralistic. When she would try to talk to him he would go on a binge; when he would try to talk to her, she would give him a sermon on the sins of his "alcoholism." By the time I saw them they had each retained lawyers for divorce proceedings. I saw them individually and then brought them together for a "go" at it. It was a memorable session. Accusations, insults, bitter invectives, near actual blows, and several moves by each partner to leave the session ensued. However, since neither was willing to leave the battlefield to the other, both stayed until the bitter end. It managed to clear the air and allow each some consideration for the other. In relatively few succeeding sessions, the woman was able to face her fears of the menopause, causing her to fear loss of femininity, she became more understanding of her husband's somewhat similar fears of aging, and a reestablishment of the relationship followed.

I cannot overemphasize the importance the doctor has to the patient, especially if he has cared for her, and probably her family, over a long period of time. His active influence can often get the patient to modify her whole pattern of living and direct her energies into new activities. Not only does it take a psychiatrist time to develop a working relationship with a patient, but often our words are heeded less than his who has successfully coped with her past illnesses. There are a certain number of patients for whom referral to a psychiatrist is indicated: the very depressed, the psychotic, and those who do not respond well to your therapy or who you feel would benefit from more intensive psychological work. Consultation on your problem cases, I feel, could be used much more freely than it has been, and too, there should be more working together on the psychosomatic problems.

Certain patients will still have to be treated with drugs or EST, but there is a large group who will respond very well to psychotherapy. Formerly, intensive, reconstructive, or analytic therapy was considered indicated only in the younger ages. This I do not believe. Many people engaged in this last major identity crisis can use intensive therapy to resolve old conflicts and rework inefficient defenses in such manner as to reach a higher level of integration than they had ever had. An example of this would be a forty-five-year-old woman whom I first saw on consultation in the hospital. Her complaints were physical: disabling backaches, weakness, headaches and some vaso-vegetative symptoms. Underlying the symptoms was a severe depression, chronic in nature, but more intense since the cessation of her menses a year previously. She was semi-alcoholic, constantly at odds with her husband, had withdrawn from her friends, and harbored a pervasive resentment underneath an exterior of ingratiating compliance. She responded well to psychotherapy and as her physical symptoms improved she was able to resume her work. It soon became evident that her life adjustment had long been unsatisfactory and the menopause had only intensified her sense of inner frustration, bitterness, guilt and worthlessness, resulting in her total disability and hospitalization. She decided to undergo psychoanalysis and was able to resolve a severe neurosis having at its roots the death of her father when she was seven and an intensely ambivalent, guilt-ridden relationship with her mother. Today she is free of symptoms, productive in her work, active socially, and more content than she has even been. I think this case tends to demonstrate that intensive therapeutic work can be done in depth with resulting characterological changes during this period.

I have attempted in this paper to survey some of the multiple factors leading to major difficulties during the menopause. It is a complex period with stress from cultural, biological, and individual psychological spheres. Its resolution means reorganization and reorientation of psychic energies along lines more appropriate to the change in status and function. This, I believe, is a true developmental stage in the life cycle, necessitating reintegration of the personality for continuing successful adaptation. A variety of factors can enhance the difficulty in coping with this period, but of primary importance is the past success of the woman's identification with and fulfillment of her feminine role, both maternally and sexually. A past development that fosters rebellion against or inhibition of this role makes a more difficult menopause.

The frequency of depression and some of the more common pathological reactions have been mentioned and some broad therapeutic suggestions have been offered. The importance of psychotherapeutic intervention has been stressed.

Most of these problems, as in the past, will continue to be effectively handled by doctors other than psychiatrists. I hope, however, that this program emphasized a spirit of increased cooperation and communication between us in our continuing attempt to more effectively treat this difficult developmental stage.

REFERENCES

1. Benedek, T.: *Psychosexual Functions in Women*. New York, Ronald, 1952.
2. Fessler, L.: The psychopathology of climacteric depression. *Psychoanal. Quart. XIX*:28-42, 1950.

MAINTENANCE OF SUPPORTIVE CONTACT IN SCHIZOPHRENIC PATIENTS

WILLIAM S. WIEDORN, M.D.

T HE TITLE OF this paper is somewhat of a misnomer, for indeed all medical contact is supportive. Any nonsupportive contact is by definition antitherapeutic, and so will be excluded from our consideration here. We will also not concern ourselves with the questions pertaining to making the diagnosis of the occurrence of a schizophrenic illness. The assumption is that we are all in agreement as to what constitutes a schizophrenic illness and are equally in agreement as to the diagnostic criteria, though this of course is not the case.

Any physician, regardless of specialty, with an active practice sees many schizophrenic patients in his office. Patients come with any complaint—real, imagined or psychosomatic. Many schizophrenic persons are probably never diagnosed as such. Most schizophrenic persons do not get into mental hospitals or see psychiatrists. Whether they should is a moot question. If they did, they would overwhelm out-patient or in-patient psychiatric facilities by their sheer numbers. Figures vary depending on the manner in which they are obtained, but it would be fair to estimate that between 2 and 5 per cent of the population would be labelled as schizophrenic by most psychiatrically trained diagnosticians. If the criteria of some schools of thought were followed, the numbers would be even greater, and even greater than that if the so-called "borderline psychotics" were included. Further, some psychiatrists would say that many schizophrenic persons never experience a psychotic episode, in the sense of acute and severe intra-psychic disorganization becoming a social issue through severely disordered behavior. Thus we are focusing our attention here on a much broader based group than simply those patients who have been released from a mental hospital with the diagnosis: schizophrenic reaction.

Many papers written for the physician who is not a psychiatrist emphasize the difficulties in making interpersonal contact with the schizophrenic person. The patient is described as aloof, distant, easily disorganized, and given to bizarre communication. The physician is provided with a number of techniques which the author has found to be useful in dealing interpersonally with schizophrenic persons. But great caution is counselled in approaching or dealing too directly with the patient, his feelings and other psychologic activity. Perhaps this caution derives from the fact that these authors are usually psychiatrists, who traditionally do not see the schizophrenic person until after he has experienced massive and catastrophic disorganization. Various medications, labelled as "tranquilizers," but otherwise useful as sedatives of one sort or another are recommended with the hope that this will somehow make communication and contact between these two—physician and patient—more profitable and comfortable.

I shall take a different tack here and submit that the issue for the physician, as well as the schizophrenic patient, is not how to make contact, but how to avoid decreasing the intense contact that already exists. For schizophrenic persons form intense relationships with others, and are eager for contact of all kinds. This simply because they too are human and could not survive without much contact. Though we must keep in mind that the type of relationships they form and the type of contact they hunger for may not necessarily be that which has the highest statistical distribution in the community at large. Nor may it necessarily be the type of contact with which the physician is more familiar or most consciously comfortable in. An example springs readily to mind. The hostile, suspicious, paranoid schizophrenic does not make the most comfortable nor the most grateful patient for the physician to work with.

If the patient comes to the physician's office, the patient obviously wants contact. In our society, the act of a patient offering themselves to a physician for diagnosis and treatment is a literal offering of themselves for the most intimate and thorough type of contact. The patient is making a contract to tell the physician all of his innermost physical and emotional secrets, to allow him to look at and manipulate his body, both on the surface and internally, and even to allow him to take some of himself away, as with the collecting of blood, urine samples, etc. From one viewpoint there is no other type of relationship in our social structure which approaches the intimacy which is contracted for in the relationship between physician and patient, at least for the time that it exists in a treatment situation. I am emphasizing this relationship, though it is well known to all of us, in order to attempt to offset the notion that has grown up that schizophrenic persons are so difficult to communicate with. For the patient upon presenting himself to the physician is presenting himself for maximum contact and communication.

Even though we all initially agreed upon the nature of the schizophrenic illness, and even agreed upon the diagnostic criteria and techniques, I wish at this point to make a formal excursion in to classic psychiatry. The concept of the unconscious is one that is popularly well known though usually misunderstood. Structurally the unconscious of man is that segment of the human mind which is the repository of infantile, asocial, inhuman and otherwise primitive and undifferentiated drives, impulses, wishes and sought for gratifications. Further, the unconscious is the repository of all the fantasies, memories, wishes, etc., that are too painful or uncivilized for the conscious mind or social self to endure or tolerate awareness of. Much of our personality structure has to do with keeping these impulses, wishes, and memories out of our conscious awareness. If somehow these defenses were taken away, the unconscious would erupt into consciousness and the person would at that time be acutely, overtly and seriously psychotic. This of course is what happens in some toxic states, with ingestion of certain psychotomimetic drugs such as LSD or Mescaline®, and during acute psychotic schizophrenic episodes. A similar experience occurs in dreams, especially in nightmares, in which there is partial emergence of unconscious wishes into the dream awareness, and then into the waking consciousness. All of us are familar with the nagging and persistant memory of a particularly uncomfortable or frightening dream as we go about our day's activities. In this case, we are reacting with our own anxiety to the contents of our own unconscious mind as dimly recalled through the remembered dream.

Oftentimes in our therapeutic communication with the schizophrenic patient we all react with anxiety to the nearness of the unconscious in the schizophrenic patient. In a somewhat oversimplified manner it is accurate to say that the schizophrenic illness is manifested by, among other things, a closeness of unconscious wishes and feelings to the surface. The ease with which these are communicated in the clinical situation is what allows us to say: "That person is crazy," as indeed they are. When the schizophrenic person brings himself to the physician, he brings along this aspect of himself also.

All persons, physicians or no, fear craziness, equally as they fear death. Physical death is death of the body; insanity is death of the mind. It is a terrifying notion to conceive that the mind, the self, the ego, all that which is socially and personally useful, and attractive and gratifying can be dissolved and seemingly lost forever. The physician must necessarily build defenses against the experience of anxiety engendered by closeness with death. But further, the experience thrust upon one's awareness that craziness, insanity, psychosis exists is invariably evocative of anxiety. This anxiety invariably is felt within the reality oriented areas of the personality.

The schizophrenic patient forces this awareness on the physician. It is at this point that the possibility of decreasing communication and contact occurs. The unconscious response of the physician is to experience anxiety. What he then does will determine the course of the therapeutic interaction between himself and his patient. If the physician is able to become aware of his own anxiety, and to use his own defenses against it, then he has the opportunity for therapeutic interaction with the patient. If he does not become aware of his own anxious responses, he then is committed to a series of behaviors which will decrease communication and contact of all types between himself and his patient. Further complicating the problem is the fact that one of the misfortunes of being schizophrenic oftentimes includes a form of extreme hyperawareness or hypersensitivity to the feelings and responses of others, especially if they are negative or rejective.

If the physician does not use his own perceptions, unconscious and otherwise in understanding the nature of the evoked anxiety in his relationship with his patient, then he must do something.

Some of the paths he may use are the following. He may engage in a series of fantasies pertaining to the chemical or hereditary nature of mental illness, thus removing it from his own experience and himself. He may engage in a series of pharmacologic maneuvers with the patient, giving one or another type of sedative ("tranquilizer," "anti-psychotic" drug, etc.) in order to diminish the patient's communication. For as any one who has visited a large state psychiatric hospital can testify, a patient receiving large amounts of, for example, thorazine is less likely to say anything that will upset anyone. The physician may engage in a series of behaviors which drive the patient literally away from his office. One of these behaviors, paradoxically enough, is to become too overconcerned about psychologic phenomena in the patient. Schizophrenic persons, as all the rest of us, are hopefully always engaged in a process of attempted psychologic and emotional growth. These experiences are never smooth and are usually attended by anxiety. If the physician over-reacts, jumps in and begins doing all sorts of things, including medicating the patient, the patient will respond to the physician's anxiety and conveniently disappear.

Thus in summary, I have approached the problem of medical communication and interaction with the schizophrenic patient from another viewpoint. I have suggested that the issue is to attend to those processes which decrease the maximum contact and communication between the physician and patient. Many of the communications from the schizophrenic patient by their very nature invariably evoke anxiety in the other person. Attention to this allows the physician to not engage in antitherapeutic actions. As the physician devotes himself to increasing his awareness of his own perceptions, he observes increasing comfort within himself.

PANEL DISCUSSION

MODERATOR: T. A. WATTERS

PANELISTS: GALLANT, BURDON, SVENSON, AND WIEDORN

Dr. Watters:

Hope you see all this as a change in medicine, and medical education; as a new time, a new way of seeing things; a revolution—a pleasant revolution; as a stimulating revolution; as a reorientation; and finally, as a shifting of emphasis back into the area that makes man more understandable and a physician more understanding in his attempts to help them.

You've heard a rich and rewarding group of speeches this morning. I know each one of these men and their competence, and I dare say you appreciate them by this time. Now it's my task to activate the panel, to get some dissension going, to establish communication with the audience, be provocator, and have the experience point itself up with the finality that will let us leave for lunch and be happy for the experience.

I see some engaging faces in the audience. I see some who have curiosity and a few questions, but I'd like to start with the panel and say this in behalf of them. You've heard such things as Dr. Wiedorn put across this morning. This has all been, I'm sure, a wakening to you that this matter of schizophrenia isn't a dogmatic, dyed, fixed sort of thing that you read in the text books a few years ago. You've also heard Dr. Burdon and Dr. Svenson mention that anxiety is healthy. Just because someone has anxiety doesn't mean he is sick. If you didn't have anxiety, you wouldn't get going. Anxiety makes us do something. Competition is healthy. Dependency is normal, within a certain

range. Were it not for normal dependency, we wouldn't have
any friends. There would be no one we could rely on, counsel
with. It would be an isolated, lonely world. One must see these
things from a practical, relative point of view, for clinical work.

With these few remarks, I'm going to turn to the panelists and
see if I can activate some differences among them because I
know audiences well enough to know they like entertainment as
well as an opportunity for learning. I do a great deal of lecture
work in the industrial world. You wouldn't believe it, but often
they expect me to entertain as well as teach. It's a conditioned
experience for which Hollywood is remembered so faithfully and
so well. We have men on our panel who are astute clinicians,
and I'm going to begin with Dr. Burdon who may have the first
word of dissension with his fellow panelists.

Dr. Burdon:

I'll start with Dr. Wiedorn's talk. In treating schizophrenia,
he seemed to imply that chloropromazine isn't much better than
a placebo. Yet, earlier in the day, I seemed to hear Dr. Gallant
say that the NIMH, at great expense and enormous effort, had
shown that chlorpromazine, trifluoperazine and thioridazine
were a good deal better than placebos in treating schizophrenic
conditions. Notwithstanding loyalty to my friend, I would believe
the National Institute of Mental Health findings had great merit.
Perhaps the drugs might be said to *cure* the schizophrenia *but
not help* the person who happens to be the patient. Certainly
the dynamics of weak ego functioning still remain for the psychotherapist to deal with.

Dr. Gallant:

I didn't intend to present the paper this morning as anti-drug
or pro-drug. The only intention was to present some of the
available psychopharmacologic data to this audience. I mentioned mild to moderate improvement. Actually this improvement is a decrease in hallucinatory content and a decrease in
psychotic thought process. Now at that point I'm not saying
that these drugs are curing the illness. Dr. Wiedorn is of the
opinion from the therapeutic viewpoint—correct me if I'm wrong—

that it's more important to allow the patient to retain his delusional psychotic material for some time to make himself even better understood, and not to sedate the patient with some tranquilizing drug. Some psychiatrists radically disagree with this approach.

Dr. Wiedorn

Why not call them what they are, sedatives?

Dr. Gallant:

No, this is incorrect, Dr. Wiedorn. Not all antipsychotic agents have sedative action. This is an extremely important area and not only do I differ with you, but many other investigators in this area differ with you, particularly in regard to these new compounds, the Butyrophenone agents. While these compounds have definite antipsychotic activity and therapeutic efficacy in the schizophrenic population, they are almost completely lacking in sedative effects.

Dr. Watters:

Dr. Gallant, permit me to intercede. We must allow Dr. Wiedorn a chance for full rebuttal.

Dr. Gallant:

May I just add one thing about the Butyrophenone compounds. These are drugs that have almost no sedative properties. The sedation is minimal. When we compare these agents to phenobarbital which is a sedative drug, we still see a tremendous significant decrease in the psychotic symptomatology in the butyrophenone patient group as compared to the phenobarbital group (gr iii daily). Therefore, the term "sedative" would be a misleading word.

Dr. Wiedorn

Nobody, least of all me, is against short term use of a drug which dampens down symptoms and which dampens down everything else.

The only thing I'm saying is that this doesn't make somebody tranquil, it is not antipsychotic, this is not definitive treatment.

This is analagous, if you will, to giving anticough medications or antipyretics to somebody with pulmonary tuberculosis, which I think should be done. One is deluding one's self and everybody else to imply that this is in any way definitive treatment. The terms used for these medications make this implication. That's my only criticism of that.

Dr. Gallant:

I do agree with the opinion that these drugs do not "cure" schizophrenia. No one has defined schizophrenia, but I think we can all say that it's a syndrome. It's not a specific disease. All we see is a combination of symptoms and signs the patient presents. We don't know what the specific etiology is. Since we don't even know the etiology, we surely are not curing the disorder with the drug. We surely are not treating the disorder in the most specific way possible. Of that, there's no doubt.

Dr. Svenson:

I think you pay a price for everything. If you want success, you work hard. If you want to cure maladjustments in living, you've got to put an awful lot of effort into some type of psychotherapy. Other terms are short range benefits. I don't think that we can cure the underlying disease by medication. We can produce a patient whose level of function is less, but this is often a great price to pay, as far as the individual goes.

Dr. Wiedorn

Prior to the advent of the chlorpromazines, I was a first-year resident in Charity Hospital. We saw innumerable patients who would get no drugs and whose psychosis would remit in three days and they would be out in a week. We never see this in Charity Hospital now for the simple reason every patient gets slowed down and dampened down with tranquilizers, and it just takes them longer to reorganize.

Dr. Watters:

The quest for chemical magic is eternal. We have spent ten minutes on it, and I don't want it to steal the thunder. I remember the Memphis meeting of the Southern Medical Association when one panelist got off on drugs, and it was very difficult to get on anything else. Now, if we have some time left over, we'll come back to drugs. I'm not underplaying drugs. There's a great deal of important material that went across the room this morning. I think it's only fair to draw from our audience at this point and tap in on some additional thoughts. I've seen some faces eager to speak up.

Audience:

I'd like to ask Dr. Wiedorn this. Is it not usual at this time, considering the shortage of psychiatrists, that the chronic schizophrenic is usually managed by giving him chlorpromazine on a long-term basis?

Dr. Wiedorn

No, because first of all, most chronic schizophrenics are not getting drugs, because they're not being seen for treatment. And even with state hospital patients, many are not kept on long-term tranquilization.

Dr. Svenson:

There are a lot of studies which will not back you up. I think the long-term studies on chlorpromazine maintaining patients outside the hospital can't be dismissed.

They stay out of the hospitals for longer periods of time so the hospital population is decreasing probably due primarily to these drugs. Certainly there's a shortage of psychiatrists, surely there's a shortage of medical personnel to deal with these problems, a tremendous shortage. I imagine we will continue using drugs for a long period of time. However, the price we pay for it, I think, is worth consideration.

Dr. Watters:

My friend, Tom Main, in England made a study of prescription of drugs in his hospital, and it was very revealing. He found out that the drugs helped the nurses and doctors more than the patients. Again, I'm not playing down drugs. I'm simply bringing the doctor's personality in here. Drugs relieve a great deal of anxiety, often in the physician. Now my colleague to the left has a question to ask that points right up on that.

Dr. Burdon:

I wanted to take again an assertion from Dr. Wiedorn's paper. This is his insistence, which I agree with, that we physicians fear psychosis. We are afraid of psychotic processes in our patients. I would like to really discuss this oldest of all fears— to try to see if we could get a little more explanation of why this is so.

I hate to sound like a psychiatrist. The irrational, crazy, sexual, murderous, etc. impulses that all of us have as children and keep out of consciousness, out of awareness; the tremendous irrational aspects of ourselves which we fear, which erupt sometimes when we dream, when you have nightmares, etc., and which all of us know erupt sometimes when we find with idle highly anti-social fantasy. I think this is the basic fear. We fear this aspect of ourselves when somebody comes along and rubs out noses and says "Guess what." It's just a human quality.

Dr. Watters:

The desire for control increases the fear.

Audience:

Isn't it the unknown that we fear?

Dr. Burdon:

Well, if I could again act like a psychiatrist but trying to do otherwise, I would say that the unknown is given a face and given a name by us, through our own projections. Just as when you were five years old and went to sleep and saw a shadow, you knew what it was. You knew it was a rhinoceros. The unknown is known unconsciously. It's a projection of your fears.

Dr. Gallant:

Realistic anxiety can be a motivating factor for treatment. In our alcoholism clinic, if the patient was given any kind of medication at the time of his initial visit, he was unlikely to come back because his anxiety was relieved and the motivation for treatment was decreased. Our return rate for the second visit is now 89 per cent since we stopped giving medication during the first visit.

Dr. Watters:

One time I led an orchestra, and we had a fellow in it named Zivitz who played the fiddle, but when he really got going, he'd get on "E" string and we'd have to get him off. It was my painful job to get him off "E" string, so we want to get back to your question. Dr. Gallant, give us an answer to the gentleman's question about the fear of the unknown.

Dr. Gallant:

Part of the fear, I think, is a healthy fear as far as every day living is concerned. The anxiety of existence involves trying out new things that may be uncomfortable for us. A little bit of that type of anxiety is good for all of us. I think if you try to avoid this realistic anxiety you end up in a neurotic straight jacket. Our anxiety in regard to the psychotic patient is real for us. I think we should have that type of anxiety. We should learn how to accept it and tolerate it and use it in our concern for the patient. There's a possibility that some of us will have severe emotional problems at some time in the future. This, too, is going to stir us when we see somebody behaving like this right in front of our eyes.

Dr. Svenson:

The unknown is not only feared; the unknown in very anxious or very neurotic people stirs up a lot of fears because the unconscious projections are very frightening and fill up the void. However, a lot of people enjoy overcoming or mastering some of the aspects of the unknown. Why would anybody really climb a mountain or discover something new unless there was some part of them that wanted to master and experience something unknown.

Dr. Watters:

Now I think we should move to the audience and do it justice. Are there any other questions at this point?

Audience:

One of the things that comes to my mind is who are the people that come to us medically to resolve their problems, how many of these problems for others are worked out in business, in activities, in other fields which we never observe and in which the therapy, really, is an entirely different type of activity. Either the community, or the organization, or their pattern of life really treats these situations. Why do they come to us? Who are they?

Dr. Svenson:

Those who come to us are often the ones for whom the "other activities" are insufficient. For example, church is fine for many people. For some people, it isn't the answer. It breaks down someplace. It just doesn't fulfill the need, and then they have to find some other type of experience. It's the same in work. Work can be made into a kind of a straight jacket for some people by which they then can successfully avoid anxiety. It is very apt to break down along the way. It's too rigid. These people have a great amount of rigidity or inability to react flexibly toward certain types of stress.

Audience:

Speaking from the viewpoint of the internist, I would like to ask if, in all of the sessions that we have had, the overall picture that we're supposed to get is that our objective primarily is to get communication with our patient, regardless of whatever their situation, in order to have a rapport, and then, with this communication, to be able to get them to ventilate, to express themselves more and more completely—not in an effort to try to change them in any way to our way of thinking, but to bring out in themselves something substantial that has been missing so that they can have a philosophy of life or parts of a philosophy from which they can structure something within themselves which can support them in many of their minor crises, and only use drugs as a temporary tool with which to make them receptive to our effort to reach and to bring forth from them the things that we want.

Now a question to go along with this, which is confusing to me, is that many times I find if a patient has reached a severe stage of depression in which my psychiatrist friends perhaps feel that they want to use electroshock therapy, I am cautioned about using the supportive drugs because of some effect it might have on the treatment that they might want to give in a more intensive way. I wonder if there's some way of clarifying what the indications are or how fast the nonpsychiatrist should go in order to do what he's trying to do without interfering with something in the case that gets beyond him and he realizes that this is a case for referral.

Dr. Svenson:

I would answer that the treating doctor should use the best of his judgment, not worrying about what the consultant is going to say. Then when the patient gets to the consultant, he will either say, "Let me take over in this area," or "You continue in this area."

My personal experience is that though I use few drugs, if I see a patient on consultation from a general practitioner, I often like to let him handle all the drugs. Now the general practitioner can say, "I'm not going to increase your dosage. You take that up with your psychiatrist," or this type of thing.

If I use drugs, I find I eventually get into a struggle with the patient and we talk about drugs instead of talking about problems, and so I usually like the other person to handle them, if need be, and decrease them as soon as possible.

Dr. Gallant:

There are different degrees of depression that we see. The first question that comes to my mind when I'm seeing a depression is, "Is this patient also suicidal?" I would question him very specifically to see how far along this line he has gone in his thoughts and possibly his actions. If I feel he is severely suicidal,

I'd hospitalize him. I would not be adverse to using electric shock treatment. This is my own personal opinion with that particular type of patient.

On the other hand, if this is a mildly to moderately depressed person who is still functioning in his environment, I would be hesitant to use drugs. The antidepressant medications have questionable therapeutic efficacy at this time. If the patient shows satisfactory progress in psychotherapy, he might give credit to the drug instead of being able to give credit to himself. Depressed patients have a lot of magic going for them, and if you add a drug to the regimen when it's not necessary, they'll attribute their improvement to the magic of a drug instead of to themselves.

Audience:

This business about a person dying. You know they're going to die . . . Do you tell them they're going to die?

Dr. Watters:

Let's ask some members of the audience about this. I think we have some very skilled craftsmen here.

Audience:

Well, my experience before I turned psychiatrist was with children. One thing I had heard from my older general practitioner relatives turned out to be quite true, even for children as young as five years old, which is kind of shattering to the doctor, that is, that instinct does tell them they are going to die. They handle it with as great or more calm than anyone around them, including the doctor, as a rule. If you identify with children, of course, it's especially hard for a five, six or ten year old to say calmly, "You know, I'm going to die," and you to agree with them. It's much better if you can, Lord knows. I think, from our limited experience with adult medical problems, if you just listen and don't get too upset they will tell you what they know and give you a hint as to how much they want to know about it.

Dr. Watters:

Let's move it back to the panel. We have just a few minutes.

Dr. Burdon:

Well, I would say that with regard to impending death, first of all that it's more often known and suspected and "smelled in the air" than actually overtly discussed by the patient or his family. One of the first things we, as physicians, must do is to sense the emotional climate of the family, especially the spouse. I wouldn't tell the moribund member of the family that he's about to die without the family's permission and full cooperation. When I talked to you about psychiatric emergencies, I indicated they were all family-based. I think a relative's dying is an emergency of the deepest sort where intense and desperate anxiety is present, and where the job is to make the inevitable as human and humane as possible. The decision to tell of the impending death is often *post hoc;* they often know the fact already, but have not squarely faced it. You know, there's all kinds of knowing—there's knowing and not knowing, there's knowing and not telling. If you have a problem about it, it's individual and discuss it with the family. It seems to me that the physican's objective is to achieve as graceful and loving a mood of all concerned at the time of death—for some persons it is better to know all; for others, it is artful to be reassuring and hopeful to the end.

Dr. Svenson:

Most people, I think, want to know so they can go ahead and make their plans. Some patients don't want to know and I think it's a mistake to tell them. They should know whatever they need to carry on. It's an individual thing, and most often they will indicate what they want.

Audience:

I'll restrict myself to one question which I will toss up for any panelist to catch. It's two observations that seem mutually exclusive. I think they really aren't. One was that, in my pediatric years, pointing out an emotional problem and recommending psychiatric consultation, let alone therapy, turned out to be a real fine way to keep my practice from getting overloaded. It thinned it out very nicely.

Then something else. When I turned into a psychiatrist I learned, also not from the books, the therapeutic value of telling a patient either acutely or chronically schizophrenic bluntly, "You, friend, are not nervous, depressed, overworked, or anything. You are crazy."

Dr. Wiedorn

People a little crazy always know they're crazy, and they know it sooner, better, and quicker than anybody around them, including the psychiatrist.

Audience:

I'm a pediatrician. I'm not sure but what I understood that drugs, to an adolescent, were definitely harmful and that they'd stop their growth. Am I right or wrong?

Dr. Gallant:

That has never been described as any side effect of any of the psychophramacological drugs.

Dr. Watters:

It becomes my pleasure, as moderator, to bring to an end this stimulating panel, and to point up the practical remarks that came forth in our discussion. They bring us a new orientation and approach to the emotionally disturbed person. We now see him from a vantage point that makes our task less fearsome to us, and more inviting and challenging to the physician. With an acceptance of him like any other patient, and with drugs, and with mental tools to use, our chances to be helpful are multiplied. Yet, with a realization that the whole man stands before us, we can approach him with the same attitude that our antecedents did, when medicine made its first beginnings as a discipline in its own right. In a way, we are back at Epidauros.

EPILOGUE

PSYCHIATRY TODAY: ITS TRANSITIONAL STATE

WILLIAM R. SORUM, M.D.

T HE ORIGINS OF psychiatry, the oldest of the healing arts, are shrouded in the distant past. As Ehrenwald (1) has noted, psychiatry arose from certain concepts created by man: magic, which reflects his quest for omnipotence; religion, which indicates his need for salvation; and science, which represents his need for knowledge and mastery. These origins of psychiatry are still evident. We see this desire for magical results in all forms of medical practice. As for the religious need deeply embedded in the nature of man, many people consider psychiatry an answer. Finally, we like to think of ourselves as scientists, although we may not yet be. Until about two hundred years ago, mental illness was explained by demonology, and something of this idea is still evident in parlor conversations, comic strips, movies, and other media of communication.

Partly as a result of these origins, psychiatrists range in public opinion from bastard child to prodigal son; we are called charlatans by some (the radical right or left, neither of whom like us very much) and supermen by others (those who consider us omniscient). There is the judge who calls and says, "I want to get this patient to you right away because I know you can help him." He is unaware of the long standing nature of the patient's disorder and the improbability of overnight relief. Most of our critics contend that psychiatrists have delusions of omnipotence but insufficient knowledge. Perhaps it is bewildering to see a group of psychiatrists, presumably in possession of truth,

213

engaging in lively controversies most of the time, but in an emerging, dynamic speciality this is a sign of health. All fields have their controversies but because of its capacity for making people uncomfortable, psychiatry seems to be singled out for criticism of its dissension within the profession.

Like all medicine, psychiatry is in a state of transition. We cannot predict what this specialty will be like ten years from now because of changing sociocultural factors, plans for community health programs, invasion or assistance (depending on one's point of view) of the private sphere by the public domain, and transformation of psychiatric services. People who cannot afford the traditional forms of treatment need to be reached. Certainly psychoanalytic medicine, as practiced in the past, is inadequate for many people. Whereas psychiatry is being revolutionized and may be unrecognizable a decade from now, certain truths will always apply to the human being. It is here that the real value of psychiatry lies.

Psychiatry offers a unique way of looking at the individual. This specialty, more than any other, has given medicine an approach to the idea of *total man*. Admittedly, psychiatrists are not alone in using this approach, but more than most other physicians they recognize that illness is experienced at all levels of behavior—that of cells, tissues, organs, organ systems, and the whole organism, as well as that of man in relation to society. Whereas the psychiatrist must be concerned with scientific explanations for behavior, this is insufficient. He must also be concerned with alleviation of human suffering experienced in the total sphere of behavior.

Many have made contributions to the philosophy of medicine which psychiatrists follow: Claude Bernard's classic discussion of homeostasis; Cannon's work on bodily changes associated with fear of pain and rage; Sherrington's concept of the mind as manager of muscle. Freud focused attention on the unconscious mind and its often unperceived influences and the emerging patterns in men's lives that are often unrecognized. He also proposed the concept of psychic determinism, in which all acts have meaning. These insights into human behavior are not only important to psychiatrists and all physicians, but their influence is evident throughout the culture.

Psychoanalytic contributions have been numerous. As the main core of the dynamic ideas that makes psychiatry more than a descriptive discipline, psychoanalysis, has given birth to modern psychodynamic psychiatry and continues to nourish it. The tendency to restrict this knowledge and limit its availability is regrettable; therapists for emotionally or mentally ill persons must come not only from psychiatry but from medicine as a whole.

We cannot afford to permit stasis in our specialty, or withdrawal into cliques, or promulgation of rigid doctrines. It is time for relaxation of the doctrinal approach and for grasping of the opportunity to learn from other disciplines, such as anthropology, sociology, and psychology. The behaviorists, for example, are making many useful contributions despite their shortcomings. We need to learn from many people in many fields, even from philosophers and religionists, who have dealt with human illness throughout history. We must use all the knowledge available in answering the needs of patients.

Forms of therapy are continually changing. The one-to-one relationship of psychiatrist-patient is breaking down because the method of treating one patient's problems in four or five sessions each week for four or five years is often impractical for many reasons. The idea may not be entirely false that the more highly trained the psychiatrist, the less useful he is. He often retreats into forms of practice that reach only a limited segment of the population, and he may restrict his lines of communication to fellow psychiatrists. During his training, however, he deals with all types of patients, in collaboration with other doctors. While building his practice, he makes himself available to meet the needs of other doctors. Once he attains a certain status, unfortunately he is often tempted to limit his sphere of influence. The psychiatrist must re-enter the general population, extend his influence, and develop new and diversified forms of treatment. The need exists for supportive therapy in addition to reconstructive therapy.

In the past, the gulf between doctors who favored the analytic approach in psychiatry and those who favored the direct approach was almost unbridgeable. Today *all* doctors must understand the indications for both approaches in intelligent referral. The nature of modern psychiatry makes it desirable for the psychiatrist to have the broadest possible approach with multiple tools at his command for treating patients. As psychiatrists differ in varying degree from one another, so the tools which they use will vary from the suggestive approach used by all practitioners, to the far-reaching attempts at alteration of character structure used by the psychoanalytically oriented.

Of the available tools the most valuable is psychotherapy whose spectrum ranges from the supportive, through the reconstructive type of therapy. Supportive therapy which attempts with the use of suggestion, reassurance, manipulation, and guidance, to strengthen the individual's existing defenses enabling him to regain an equilibrium, includes therapy with limited insight as well as the re-educative type. Reconstructive therapy, considered the province of the psychoanalyst, seeks to give the individual an insight into unconscious conflicts, thus altering his character structure extensively, enabling him to develop new adaptive potentials.

Some years ago, in the book *Social Class and Mental Illness* (2) an interesting study was made of the relationship of the practice of psychiatry to the social structure. This study sought to point out that practitioners could be separated into two groups, the analytical-psychological and the direct-organic. The A-P group specialized largely in intensive psychotherapy, limiting themselves to the purely psychological approach while minimizing the use of drugs and organic therapy. The D-O group on the other hand, priding themselves on their "common-sense approach," used an almost exclusively organic therapy. Tranquilizers along with other drugs, and electric-shock therapy were in large measure the only tools on which they depended. As in any grouping of this nature the individuals varied with some overlapping in the degree to which they fit the category.

This study went on to point out that if patients were divided into five general classes according to their place in the social structure, the first two, or upper classes, would be largely the province of the analytical-psychological practitioner. The remaining classes, the lower two-thirds of the population, would not be considered good cases for psychological treatment, and would be the province of the direct-organic practitioner. Thus it becomes evident; not only are psychiatrists divided in their thinking and practice, but the social class and financial means of the patient determine to a large extent the treatment which they receive.

This book had a tremendous impact. In recent years, however, there has been a tendency to move away from the situation which it pointed out. There is an increasing integration of approaches used, with application to all segments of the population of a more flexible, broad-spectrum psychotherapy. Many authorities, having observed the trends in psychiatric practice, see a gradual blurring of the line of demarcation between dynamic psychotherapy and formal psychoanalysis. This may serve to abolish the class distinctions which have arisen in psychiatry.

Flexibility of approach, which allows the needs of the patient to determine the type of therapy which he will receive, is of great importance. Present day medical education seeks to produce a competent psychotherapist who can do long-term intensive psychotherapy as well as modified supportive therapy; or variations in between as they are appropriate. This flexibility is possible without destroying the basic psychoanalytic doctrine, and with preservation of psychodynamic and psychoanalytic insights. It can be the outgrowth of searching examination of older doctrines, and awareness of new trends in therapeutic approach. These might be generally accepted trends such as group therapy, family therapy (treating the family as a unit), and revolutionary methods of hospital treatment; or these might be interesting trends in therapy which are presently beyond the mainstream of current psychiatric practice, for example, the rational therapy of Albert Ellis, or the reality therapy of Glasser.

Additional tools for the therapist are to be found among the specialized techniques aimed primarily at symptom removal, which claim to be more far-reaching in effect than mere supportive measures. One example is Wolpe's reciprocal inhibition therapy which uses suggestion and hypnosis in the process of conditioning. There has been a proliferation of these conditioning techniques, partly in response to the ever-present reaction against psychoanalytic ideas.

Many physicians are aware of the chemotherapeutic revolution which is taking place in psychiatry. More and more drugs are available which, if not the universal panaceas promised by some magazines and drug companies, have proved to be strongly useful adjuncts to psychotherapeutic treatment of patients. Though some practitioners seem to feel that chemotherapeutic control of anxiety and suppression of psychotic symptomology is sufficient, the best use of drugs is in conjunction with other types of therapy. No patient should be denied the benefit of carefully prescribed drugs while the practitioner relies solely on psychotherapeutic techniques, nor should the patient have to depend on drugs alone. An either/or approach should be avoided. Electro-shock therapy has been greatly modified by the use of drugs. While it is still a valid form of treatment, the need for it has lessened considerably. In a hospital where formerly twenty-five to thirty treatments in a day would not be unusual, the number is now down to five or less.

Other changes which lie ahead for psychiatric practice will grow out of an increasing emphasis on community mental health programs. Large, remote hospitals will gradually be replaced by community centers providing in-patient and out-patient treatment, with facilities for day care or night care as needed. These centers will work constructively with local social agencies and medical personnel. As part of these community programs, preventive psychiatry which would seek out and attempt to eliminate causes of mental illness could become a reality.

One serious problem in our specialty today is that persons who have had no training in psychiatry are experimenting with treatment. Psychologists want to be therapists. There is a national association of ministers who are attempting to carry out so-called analytic therapy without supervision from medical sources. Even the social worker with a nodding acquaintance with the Freudian approach wants to be a therapist. Whereas many therapists are needed to take care of all the patients with mental and emotional disorders, treatment should be given only under qualified medical supervision. More physicians should learn to provide psychiatric advice to their patients rather than refer every problem, no matter how trivial, to the specialist. Often the problem can be better understood by the attending physician, and psychiatric referral is unnecessary. It is unfortunate that in many mental health clinics, social workers and psychologists are handling most of the therapy, the psychiatrist having been relegated to administration.

Several points deserve emphasis in the handling of patients. We should avoid becoming slaves to labels and classifications. Classification can be helpful but not if it governs and limits our treatment and expectations. In my early days of psychiatric training, residents had the regrettable tendency to learn labels, apply them, and thus determine treatment. Psychiatric training has improved greatly since that time, with a shift of emphasis to more dynamic learning, but in former years a conference of first-year residents might result in a vote of six to five that a patient was schizophrenic and therefore therapeutically hopeless. Or the decision might be that the patient was organically ill and therefore amenable only to organic treatment, with disregard for the fact that all illness is both psychic and organic and should be treated accordingly.

Another point that is often overlooked is that patients are human beings, members of the community, and as Erich Fromm has said, should be given the privilege of participating creatively as much as possible in his community. These patients become "cured" as their identity as human beings and members of society is restored. The use of the word *cured* here is, of course, based on a dynamic rather than a static view of life.

Concern with man as a value-seeking animal will always be important to doctors, as long as our society remains free. As important as the instinct for sex is the need for personal values. The psychiatrist's role here is not to impose values on his patients, but to enable the patient to remove the internal and external barriers that prevent him from making his own judgments.

Psychiatry is not a way of life. As a novice in the field about twenty years ago, I had almost unrealistic expectations of psychiatry as a means of self-control and self-improvement and as a solution to neuroses. I have learned that although it does not provide the meaning for human existence, psychiatry makes one aware of his need for meaning in life. It follows from this recognition that man has at least some capacity for free choice. I cannot therefore agree with B. F. Skinner (3) that "The hypothesis that man is not free is essential to the application of scientific method to the study of human behavior." Nor do I concur with the Austrian sociologist, Ludwig Gumplowicz (4), who believes that "The great error of individualistic psychology is the supposition that man thinks. . . . The individual simply plays the part of the prism which receives the rays, dissolves them according to fixed laws and allows them to pass out again in a predetermined direction and with predetermined colors." These ideas negate any possible therapeutic help for patients beyond adjustment to a fatalistic philosophy of life.

For our work to be meaningful we must believe that man has definite, if limited, freedom of choice. If we do, we can present him with the possible choices—choices that would enable him to be a creative person, a person who can relate satisfactorily to others, who can love, participate socially with others and have a commitment to value beyond himself. Without imposing our own values on anyone, we must continue to try to restore the person to his own choices, proper use of his creativity, and to participation in a democratic society.

REFERENCES

1. Ehrenwald, J.: *From Medicine Man to Freud.* New York, Dell, 1956, p. 17.
2. Hollingshead, A. B., and Redlich, F. C.: *Social Class and Mental Illness.* New York, John Wiley and Sons, Inc., 1958.
3. Skinner, B. F.: cited by Matson, F. W.: *The Broken Image.* New York, Braziller, 1964, p. 46.
4. Glumplowicz, L.: cited by Matson, F. W.: *The Broken Image.* New York, Braziller, 1964, p. 41.

AUTHOR AND DISCUSSANT INDEX

SUBJECT INDEX

A

Abdominal operations, 142 f.
Abortion, 161 f.
Accidents
  and alcoholism, 113
ACTH, 165
Adhesions, 143
Adolescence, 114 ff., 152 f, 158
Age
  and hypochondriasis, 25, 190
  and sexual behavior, 35 f., 158 ff.,
    189, 190, 191, 193
Air Force
  suicide in, 59 ff.
Alcohol, 49, 96, 100
  addiction, 78, 83
  habituation, 78 f., 83
  prescribed, 97 f.
  See also Alcoholism.
Alcoholics Anonymous, 65, 80, 105 f.
Alcoholism, 34, 36, 37, 64 f., 76 ff.,
  96 ff., 101, 103 ff., 206 f., 112, 177
  classification, 82 ff.
  and depression, 101
  drug therapy for, 170 f.
  psychological components, 77 f.
  treatment, 79, 83 f.
  See also Alcohol.
Ambivalence, 92
Amenorrhea, 87 f.
Amphetamines, 184 f.
Anger
  and hypochondriasis, 23, 25, 26
  and suicide, 59
Anorectal surgery, 143
Anorexia, 87
Antabuse®, 102

Antianxiety drugs, 169 f. *See also*
  specific agents.
Antidepressants, 94 f., 166 ff., 184
  in alcoholism, 84
  See also specific agents.
Antipsychotic drugs, 165 f., 203f.
  See also specific agents.
Anxiety, 34 f., 72, 86 ff., 173 f., 178 f.,
  201, 206 ff.
  in adolescence, 117, 119
  in alcoholism, 82, 96, 97 f.
  drug therapy for, 168, 196 f.
  and menopause, 191
  in physician, 199 f.
  and placebos, 165
  and surgery, 142
Appendectomy, 143
Appointments, 13
Asceticism
  in adolescence, 123
Asthma, 143

B

Barbiturates, 95, 169
Behavioral changes, 36 ff.
Boston City Hospital
  alcoholism research, 76 ff.
Brain
  acute syndromes, 177
  disease, 37 f.
Butyrophenone compounds, 166, 203

C

Cancer
  and suicide, 176
Carbohydrate metabolism, 49 f.